1·4·78

Glaucoma Guidebook

Glaucoma
Guidebook

GERALD L. PORTNEY, M.D.

Late Professor and Chairman
Department of Ophthalmology
University of California, Davis

Lea & Febiger
1977
Philadelphia

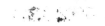

Library of Congress Cataloging in Publication Data

Portney, Gerald L
  Glaucoma guidebook.

Bibliography: p.
  Includes index.
  1. Glaucoma.   I. Title. [DNLM: 1. Glaucoma.
WW290 B853g]
RE871.P67   617.7'41   77-1568
ISBN 0-8121-0587-7

Published in Great Britain by Henry Kimpton Publishers, London

PRINTED IN THE UNITED STATES OF AMERICA

Print Number: 3   2   1

To Susan Beth,

my inspiration

and companion

PREFACE

This book is designed to serve as an introduction to glaucoma for the beginner as well as a ready reference to the many clinically relevant aspects of this disease for the more advanced. It is not intended to be an exhaustive treatise on the subject but, instead, is a vehicle oriented toward a fundamental understanding of glaucoma as a whole.

The first section, Diagnosis and Therapy, is composed of four chapters: Basic Concepts, Open-Angle Glaucomas, Angle-Closure Glaucomas, and Congenital Glaucomas. In each, the subject matter has been entirely selected to impart the essentials of patient management rather than to explore the scientific principles behind each concept in compendium fashion. In addition, the bibliography listed with each chapter has been chosen because of its critical relationship to the subject and represents mandatory reading for those who wish to obtain an in-depth perspective on glaucoma. To simplify the process, each reference has been annotated with at least one of the main thoughts conveyed by the article cited.

The second section, Clinical Examination Methods, is principally a "cook book" on the Technique of Projection Perimetry and the Stereoscopic Evaluation of the Optic Cup, its two chapters. The procedures that they describe reflect not only the personal values of the author but also include major new ideas that have been derived from recent advances in research. It is anticipated that, if the protocols described are followed fully, diagnostically useful results can be obtained every time.

In the third section, Background on Glaucoma, the chapter on The Etiology of Glaucoma: Past, Present and Future Theories, is primarily a chronology of events that have led to the present level of knowledge of the causes of glaucoma. It will provide both an overview of the subject for those with a limited interest in medical history as well as a broad foundation for those interested in the evolution of ophthalmic awareness. The Glossary is primarily oriented toward readers with limited prior exposure to general ophthalmology.

It is hoped that this book will fill an unmet educational need between that provided by purely introductory texts on glaucoma and more extensive reviews of this subject, and, by so doing, that the various practitioners involved in ophthalmic health care delivery at all levels will find their working knowledge of glaucoma significantly enhanced.

Davis, California   GERALD L. PORTNEY

ACKNOWLEDGMENTS

I would like to express my personal appreciation to Olga Raveling, who has arduously worked in the preparation of this manuscript; to Hal Pullum for his artistry; and to Francis J. Sousa, M.D., whose editorial suggestions have been of major assistance. Above all, I wish to recognize the teachings of my mentor, Peter C. Kronfeld, M.D., who showed me the meaning of glaucoma.

In addition, although I have individually reviewed and verified each reference cited here, special thanks is due to previous authors on the history of glaucoma such as Redmond J. H. Smith and Sir Stewart Duke-Elder whose writings provided valuable direction to my own investigation of the past.

CONTENTS

SECTION II
CLINICAL EXAMINATION METHODS

SECTION III
BACKGROUND ON GLAUCOMA

Glaucoma Guidebook

Section I

Diagnosis and Therapy

Chapter 1

BASIC CONCEPTS

DEFINITION OF GLAUCOMA

Glaucoma is a disease in which the intraocular pressure damages the optic nerve head. The most widely held explanation for this change is that the intraocular pressure on the peripapillary and/or intrapapillary capillaries is high enough to occlude (partially or completely) these small vessels. In so doing, the glial and nervous elements of the optic nerve head become atrophic. It is believed that, in the early stages of this oxygen deprivation, a lowering of the intraocular pressure will allow regeneration of astroglia, especially in children. Basically, according to this hypothesis, the relative difference between the external pressure upon the capillaries supplying the optic nerve head and the intracapillary pressure determines whether or not glaucoma will occur.

Alternative theories regarding the cause of damage to the optic nerve are (1) compromise of retrolaminar axoplasmic flow, or (2) a direct pressure effect on the retinal nerve fibers themselves. At this time, however, neither of these hypotheses has been proven to be true.

FACTORS RELATED TO INCREASED INTRAOCULAR PRESSURE

Intraocular pressure is determined physiologically by the relative rates of aqueous inflow and outflow. Therefore, the only possible mechanisms leading to increased intraocular pressure are increased inflow of aqueous, decreased outflow, or both. The first possibility has been virtually disregarded by most investigators as being a major problem. A few patients have been discovered who were shown to have an increased inflow, by tonographic studies, but they have been in the minority. Thus, decreased outflow is the main cause of increased intraocular pressure.

Much confusion existed in the past over the cause of this decreased outflow. In fact, it was not until 1938 that Otto Barkan put this problem into perspective. He divided glaucomatous eyes into wide-angle and narrow-angle categories. Today, these two types are referred to as open-angle glaucoma and angle-closure glaucoma.

The latter comprises those types that have an actual, physically identifiable block posterior or adjacent to the innermost trabecular sheet that prohibits the successful egress of aqueous. Open-angle glaucomatous eyes are presumed to possess an obstruction to outflow somewhere between the innermost trabecular sheet and the episcleral veins, into which the aqueous ultimately flows.

PHYSICALLY IDENTIFIABLE BLOCKS

In most cases the iris itself occludes the trabeculum. In some forms of secondary angle-closure glaucoma, the occlusion may be caused by (1) anterior synechiae, or (2) fibrous or neovascular membranes.

In both primary and secondary forms, the question of whether the initial exciting event was pupillary block is most important, and this topic will be discussed in detail under the subject of angle-closure glaucoma.

THEORETICAL BLOCKS

Some of these blocks have been identified gonioscopically, but others remain unknown. The latter group, in which there is no clinically visible obstruction, comprises the category of primary open-angle glaucoma. As will be discussed in Section

III, each of the following has been suggested at some time as a cause of this disease:

1. trabecular sclerosis
2. trabecular degeneration
3. trabecular damage
4. trabecular pigment
5. hyaluronidase
6. ciliary muscle
7. trabecular flaccidity
8. afferent arterioles
9. neurovascular reflex

Unfortunately, none of the foregoing mechanisms has been proven to be causative, so the concept of "primary" open-angle glaucoma remains alive. Recently, however, as a result of electron microscopic studies, more substantive information has emerged. These studies suggest that the site of aqueous blockade is in the endothelial meshwork at the junction of the outermost trabeculum and the inner wall of Schlemm's canal. Apparently, the fluid enters the canal almost entirely through pores in the endothelium; these channels are either associated with vacuoles or are located in the flat portion of the cells. Endothelial tubules jut into the canal of Schlemm and perhaps function as one-way tubular valves for the outflow of aqueous.

In contrast to the speculation about the cause of primary open-angle glaucoma, the etiology of secondary open-angle glaucoma is relatively more clear. The following are most of the known general categories:

1. inflammatory
2. traumatic
3. neovascular-hemolytic
4. syndrome-related
    a. pigmentary dispersion
    b. (pseudo) exfoliation

SUGGESTED READINGS

Anderson, D. R.: Pathogenesis of glaucomatous cupping: A new hypothesis. *In* Symposium on Glaucoma, 23rd, 1974: Transactions of the New Orleans Academy of Ophthalmology. pp. 81-94. St. Louis, C.V. Mosby Co., 1975. (Extensive review of conflicting theories.)

————: Pathology of the glaucomas. Brit. J. Ophthalmol. 56:146-157, 1972. (Synechiae are actually the fibrous scar tissues that provide the "cement" for the production of permanent iridocorneal adhesions.)

Becker, B., Keskey, G. R., and Christensen, R.E.: Hypersecretion glaucoma. Arch. Ophthalmol. 56:180-187, 1956. (This unusual cause of glaucoma is detected by finding an elevation of pressure without an attendant reduction in outflow.)

Grant, W. M.: Clinical measurements of aqueous outflow. Arch. Ophthalmol. 46:113-131, 1951. (The first detailed report on the measurement of the coefficient of outflow in a wide variety of glaucomatous diseases.)

Hayreh, S. S.: Optic disc changes in glaucoma. Brit. J. Ophthalmol. 56:175-185, 1972. (The sole vascular support to the optic disc is from the ciliary circulation, which is highly susceptible to compromise from elevated intraocular pressure.)

Henkind, P.: New observations on radial peripapillary capillaries. Invest. Ophthalmol. 6:103-108, 1967. (The destination of this retinal capillary system is the layer of nerve fibers that arises from the arcuate area around the macula; their loss could cause a Bjerrum scotoma.)

Johnstone, M. A.: Pressure-dependent changes in configuration of the endothelial tubules of Schlemm's canal. Am. J. Ophthalmol. 78:630-638, 1974. (Tubules project into the lumen of Schlemm's canal and become patent when the intraocular pressure rises.)

Schulze, R. R.: Rubeosis iridis. Am. J. Ophthalmol. 63:487-495, 1967. (A neovascular membrane forms by the simultaneous growth of minute blood vessels and mesenchymal cells; it occurs in many conditions which can be lumped into vascular, retinal, and iris disease categories.)

Tripathi, R. C.: Aqueous outflow pathway in normal and glaucomatous eyes. Brit. J. Ophthalmol. 56:157-174, 1972. (Discussion of macropinocytosis of the trabecular endothelium with human electron microscopic examples of the vacuolization process.)

Chapter 2

OPEN-ANGLE GLAUCOMAS

DIAGNOSTIC CONSIDERATIONS

The signs of open-angle glaucoma are:

1. increased intraocular pressure
2. visual field loss
3. optic nerve head atrophy
4. gonioscopically open angles
5. positive provocative tests
6. decreased facility of outflow

Intraocular Pressure Level

Increased intraocular pressure has various interpretations. Although 97.5% of normal individuals are believed to have pressures of 21 mm Hg or less, no one can say that "below a specific pressure the optic nerve head is safe." Furthermore, a small group of patients sustain glaucomatous damage even with pressures under 20 mm Hg. Under ordinary circumstances, one should be suspicious of pressure readings in the high twenties and be seriously concerned about those in the thirties or greater. If a patient over 50 years of age consistently has pressures of 30 mm Hg or above even without visual field loss, one should probably initiate treatment because of the likelihood that the generally decreased vascular perfusion of older people can endanger the optic nerve. In a younger patient with similar pressure readings, it may be necessary only to evaluate the optic disc and visual fields at specific intervals.

Because the Schiøtz tonometer alone is not sufficiently precise to be reliable under all clinical conditions, applanation tonometry is the method of choice for monitoring all patients except those who are particularly uncooperative. The basic reason for the inconsistency of Schiøtz tonometry is that it is based on the principle of corneal indentation. That is, the tonometer preset weight is applied to the cornea, the plunger indents it to an extent that depends on the ability of the cornea and intraocular pressure to withstand such indentation, and a scale reading, not the pressure, is read from the instrument. Unfortunately, because of individual dissimilarities in scleral rigidity, the amount of corneal indentation may vary even when the exact same weight is applied and the exact same intraocular pressure opposes the indentation. The true ocular tension is then calculated by approximating the area of indentation and applying a standard physics formula to obtain the actual pressure measurement. These calculations have been made on a number of occasions. At the present time, Schiøtz tonometry uses the results of the 1955 calibration, from which the instrument scale reading is converted directly into millimeters of mercury (Table 2–1).

On the other hand, Goldmann applanation tonometry always causes a constant area of flattening (3.06 mm diameter), no matter how high or low the intraocular pressure. The ocular tension is then calculated by measuring the exact amount of force required to perfectly flatten the cornea. Although there is some corneal resistance to deformation with this instrument, this resistance is balanced exactly by the tendency of the tears to attract the tonometer to the cornea. The measurement procedure is performed at the slit lamp, where fluorescein is placed in the patient's eye to make the tear film more apparent and an anesthetic is used to reduce corneal sensation. A conoid, flat-tipped instrument with a transparent center is pressed up against the cornea, while the

Table 2-1. Calibration Scale for Schiøtz Tonometers, P_0 (mm Hg), Revised 1955.

Scale Reading	Plunger Load			
	5.5 gm	7.5 gm	10.0 gm	15.0 gm
0.0	41.4	59.1	81.7	127.5
0.5	37.8	54.2	75.1	117.9
1.0	34.5	49.8	69.3	109.3
1.5	31.6	45.8	64.0	101.4
2.0	29.0	42.1	59.1	94.3
2.5	26.6	38.8	54.7	88.0
3.0	24.4	35.8	50.6	81.8
3.5	22.4	33.0	46.9	76.2
4.0	20.6	30.4	43.4	71.0
4.5	18.9	28.0	40.2	66.2
5.0	17.3	25.8	37.2	61.8
5.5	15.9	23.8	34.4	57.6
6.0	14.6	21.9	31.8	53.6
6.5	13.4	20.1	29.4	49.9
7.0	12.2	18.5	27.2	46.5
7.5	11.2	17.0	25.1	43.2
8.0	10.2	15.6	23.1	40.2
8.5	9.4	14.3	21.3	38.1
9.0	8.5	13.1	19.6	34.6
9.5	7.8	12.0	18.0	32.0
10.0	7.1	10.9	16.5	29.6
10.5	6.5	10.0	15.1	27.4
11.0	5.9	9.1	13.8	25.3
11.5	5.3	8.3	12.6	23.3
12.0	4.9	7.5	11.5	21.4
12.5	4.4	6.8	10.5	19.7
13.0	4.0	6.2	9.5	18.1
13.5		5.6	8.6	16.5
14.0		5.0	7.8	15.1
14.5		4.5	7.1	13.7
15.0		4.1	6.4	12.6
15.5			5.8	11.4
16.0			5.2	10.4
16.5			4.7	9.4
17.0			4.2	8.5
17.5				7.7
18.0				6.9
18.5				6.2
19.0				5.6
19.5				4.9
20.0				4.5

(From Friedenwald, J. S.: Tonometer calibration. Trans. Am. Acad. Ophthalmol. Otolaryngol. 61:108–123, 1957.)

observer sights through the double prism in its shaft. There he sees two semicircles of fluorescent tear film which he moves so that they just interlock, by adjusting the pressure on the cornea with a micrometer (Fig. 2–1). The end point on the micrometer scale of this tonometer can be converted directly into millimeters of mercury by multiplying by ten. The applanation form of pressure measurement is more accurate because it does not depend on variations in scleral rigidity nor on determining the volume of corneal indentation, a quantity that, at best, can only be approximated in each individual.

Abnormal keratometry readings may affect the reliability of the Goldmann applanation readings. For example, when the cornea is edematous, scarred, or irregular, distortion of the fluorescent images makes them difficult, if not impossible, to read. Experimentation done under these same conditions indicates that the Schiøtz readings do not correlate well with simultaneous anterior chamber manometry.

In contrast to these two instruments, the MacKay-Marg tonometer gives excellent results. It is designed on the applanation principle, but uses a centrally located plunger-transducer that senses the ocular tension. It is not affected by the surface tension of the tears or corneal resistance, as is the Goldmann device. Its readings are reliable only if the graphic

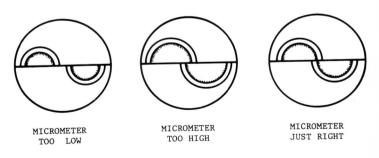

MICROMETER
TOO LOW

MICROMETER
TOO HIGH

MICROMETER
JUST RIGHT

Fig. 2-1.   Appearance of fluorescent semicircles seen through the prisms of the Goldmann applanation tonometer.

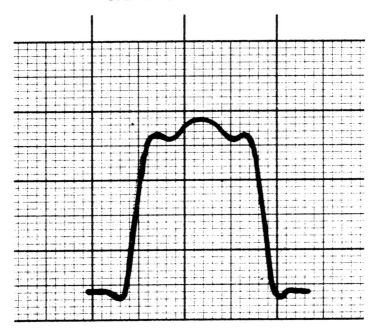

Fig. 2-2. Appearance of a "good" tracing made with the MacKay-Marg applanation tonometer.

readings can be characterized as "good" (Fig. 2–2). On normal corneas, these readings are consistently a few millimeters higher than Goldmann readings. The newer digital version of this instrument has the disadvantage of not providing a tracing for the tonometrist to evaluate.

Other portable applanation tonometers, such as the Halberg and the Draeger or Perkins, also give accurate results. Beginners may find the former instrument easier to learn, while experienced ophthalmologists may prefer the latter owing to its similarities with the Goldmann tonometer.

Visual Field Testing Devices

Visual field loss is a directly determined but subjective psychophysical measurement. Consistency of examination technique and an intimate knowledge of the perimetric instrument being used are, therefore, of utmost importance.

Tangent Screen. This remains the most common and most usable of all devices. Either a one- or two-meter screen may be used, the latter having the advantage of greater flexibility in testing. The target may be either self-luminous or a white pin on the end of a wand. The only crucial requirement is that it be possible to remove the target from view without removing the wand; for this purpose, a retractable pin is best. In testing for early glaucomatous defects with a one-meter screen, the patient should be seated at a distance of one meter in front of the screen. Unless the visual acuity is so reduced as to require a larger one, the initial target should be 2 mm in diameter and white. The notation for this testing is 2/1000, which expresses the target diameter in the numerator and the testing distance in the denominator, both in millimeters. An even illumination of 7 foot-candles on the screen is required and should be calibrated frequently with a light meter. Finally, the patient should wear his refractive correction for a one-meter distance and his fixation should be constantly monitored.

Goldmann Perimeter. This device is known as a projection perimeter; it is a half sphere in which the patient places his head during testing with projected targets. His fixation is monitored through a viewing telescope behind the perimeter; from this location the target is moved by an accurate and sensitive pantographic mechanism. As with tangent screen perimetry, proper refractive correction is essential. In addition, frequent calibration of target and background luminance (31.5 asb) is critical to the reliability of the results obtained with this machine. The perimeter is 30 cm in radius, so that the testing distance is invariant. However, both the area and luminance of the target are variable (Tables 2–2, 2–3).

Table 2-2. Target Notation and Area (mm²) on the Goldmann Perimeter.

Notation	Area
0	1/16
I	1/4
II	1
III	4
IV	16
V	64

Table 2-3. Target Filter Notation and Luminance (asb) on the Goldmann Perimeter.

Notation	e	d	c	b	a
1	31.5	25	20	16	12.5
2	100	80	63	50	40
3	315	250	200	160	125
4	1000	800	630	500	400

The size of the normal isopter varies with age, requiring greater target luminance or area to plot the same size isopter as a person ages (Table 2–4). Furthermore, because of the hole in the dome to accommodate the fixation telescope, the central 2 degrees of the visual field cannot be plotted without a special additional attachment.

Tubinger Perimeter. This projection perimeter differs from the Goldmann machine as follows: it has a background luminance of 10 asb, a radius of 33 cm, and variable size and intensity fixation points (Table 2–5); it specifies the visual angle of the target in degrees or minutes (Table 2–6); and it provides for the monitoring of fixation with a mirror system,

Table 2-4.   Nasal Radius of the Isopters for Various
Age Groups (Degrees).

Age	$I/_{1e}$	$I/_{2e}$	$I/_{3e}$	$I/_{4e}$	$II/_{4e}$
29	20	35	45	55	–
39	12	25	40	45	–
63	5	10	20	35	45

(Adapted from Haag-Streit Perimeter 940. Instructions: Assembly, Use and
Maintenance. Berne, Switzerland.)

Table 2-5.   Tubinger Perimeter Fixation Points.

Visual Angle	Luminance
10 minutes	
30 minutes	.0000016 to
1 degrees	1000 asb in
2 degrees	.2 log unit
3 degrees	steps
11 degrees	
Pericentral: 10 or 30 minutes	

Table 2-6.   Tubinger Perimeter Test Targets.

Visual Angle (minutes)	Luminance
7	
10	
17	.00001 to
26	1000 asb in
42	.1 log unit
66	steps
104	

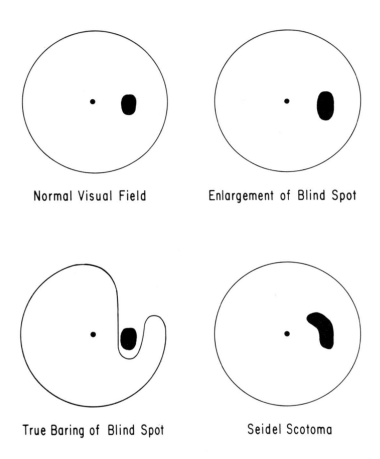

Normal Visual Field   Enlargement of Blind Spot

True Baring of Blind Spot   Seidel Scotoma

Fig. 2-5. Nonglaucomatous visual field defects.

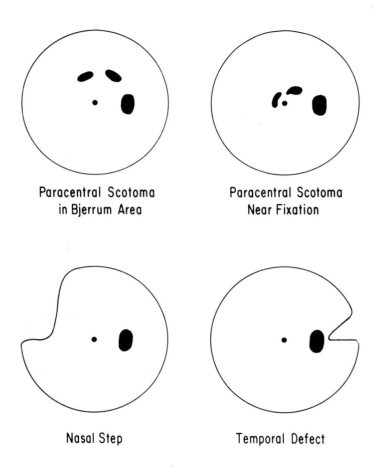

Fig. 2-6. Early glaucomatous visual field defects.

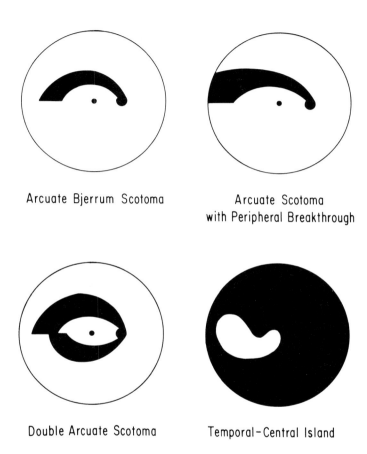

Fig. 2-7. Advanced glaucomatous visual field defects.

As glaucoma progresses, an arcuate scotoma may occur in the opposite half of the visual field. From this point, true glaucomatous field changes primarily involve a constriction of the remaining field, leaving a small central island or only a small temporal island of field or both (Fig. 2–7). Only when the central island is finally compromised does the visual acuity decrease in a glaucomatous eye.

Factors that can compromise the visual field and simulate glaucomatous change are extreme miosis, refractive error, and clouding of the media. It is crucial that the ophthalmologist be aware of their status when interpreting the results of perimetry; he must make certain that the pupil is at least 3 mm in diameter (using mydriatics for dilation if necessary) and that the refraction is correct whenever quantitiative examination is undertaken. Unless the pupil size is sufficient and the refraction proper, perimetry should be delayed until these factors are corrected.

Other ocular and neurologic problems of the anterior visual pathways can cause arcuate nerve fiber bundle defects. Among these are occlusion of a central retinal branch vein or artery, the presence of myelinated nerve fibers in the retina, optic disc drusen or pit, meningioma, pituitary adenoma, craniopharyngioma, and arachnoid cyst. Patients whose field loss is out of proportion to their optic disc damage and those who have low intraocular pressure with apparently glaucomatous visual field change should be evaluated with these diseases in mind.

Optic Nerve Head Changes

Atrophy of the optic nerve head is a subject that is complex and, as yet, incompletely defined. In order to understand it fully, a knowledge of normal or physiologic variations in the optic nerve head is necessary. Recent photogrammetric studies have begun to add an element of quantitative precision to the qualitative optic cup descriptions of the past decade. As a result of this new contour mapping technique, it

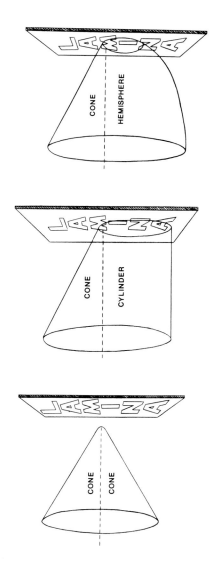

Fig. 2-8. Diagrammatic representation of cone-cone, cone-cylinder and cone-hemisphere shapes of normal optic cups.

appears that the three-dimensional shapes for normal cups tend to cluster around nine predominant geometric configurations. Three of them fit the characteristics of a cone, a cylinder or a hemisphere. Combinations of halves of these three basic geometric shapes make up the top and bottom portions of the remaining normal forms: a cone-cylinder, a cone-hemisphere, a cylinder-cone, a cylinder-hemisphere, a hemisphere-cone and a hemisphere-cylinder (Figs. 2–8, 2–9, 2–10).

Further analysis has shown that cups in which no lamina is visible before the onset of glaucoma (e.g., a cone) deepen centrally, baring the lamina early in the disease (Fig. 2–11). From this point on, the maximal depth of the cup does not significantly increase until late in the glaucomatous process. Subsequent enlargement at the bottom of the cup seems to occur by a nearly centrifugal atrophy which exposes an increasingly larger area of lamina as glaucoma advances (Fig. 2–12). A cup that has already reached the lamina in its physiologic state (e.g., cylinder) expands at its edges without undergoing initial deepening (Fig. 2–13).

In the plane of the cup orifice, the basic pattern of atrophy is one of concentrically expanding, vertically oriented ellipses (Fig. 2–14). The enlarging cup usually erodes the superior and inferior margin of the disc before completely excavating the temporal rim (Fig. 2–15). The temporal margin atrophies next, leaving the nasal tissue until the end (Fig. 2–16). Commonly, this elliptic erosion process lags in one direction and the cup extends upward and downward asynchronously (Fig. 2–17).

A far less geometrically complex system of disc evaluation is based on the concept of cup/disc ratio; that is, the determination of the approximate horizontal or vertical diameter of the cup expressed as a fraction of the diameter of the disc (Fig. 2–18). For example, such an estimate might be any number from .1 to 1.0. This method, by itself, is insufficient to fully describe a cup, but it can be a useful adjunct for chart notations when used to describe both the

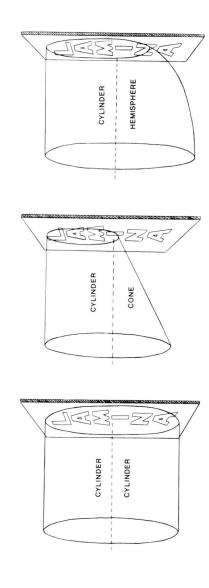

Fig. 2-9. Diagrammatic representation of cylinder-cylinder, cylinder-cone and cylinder-hemisphere shapes of normal optic cups.

25

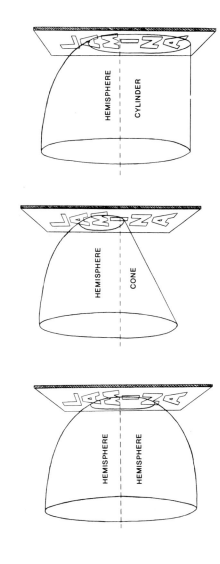

Fig. 2-10. Diagrammatic representation of hemisphere-hemisphere, hemisphere-cone and hemisphere-cylinder shapes of normal optic cups.

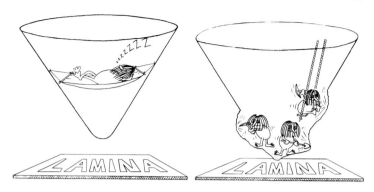

Fig. 2-11. Initial deepening of originally shallow optic cups due to glaucoma.

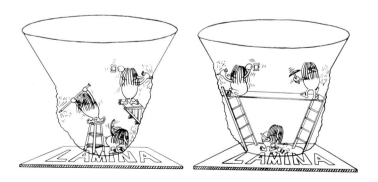

Fig. 2-12. Centrifugal enlargement at base of optic cup due to glaucoma.

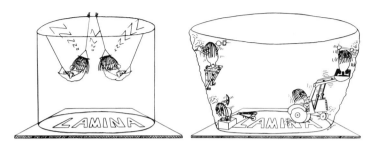

Fig. 2-13. Early circumferential destruction of the walls of originally deep optic cup due to glaucoma.

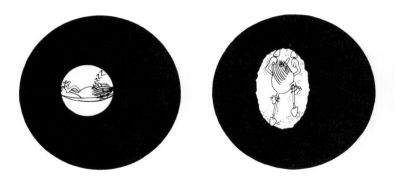

Fig. 2-14. Initial simultaneous lengthening and widening of optic cup orifice due to glaucoma.

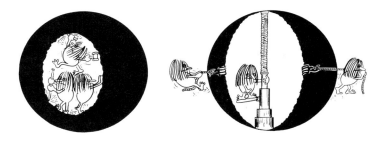

Fig. 2-15. Concentrically expanding optic cup orifice eroding superior and inferior nerve rim due to glaucoma.

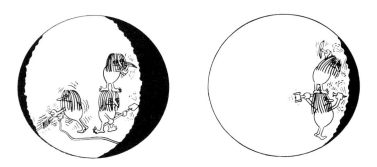

Fig. 2-16. Excavation of temporal margin of optic nerve before loss of nasal rim due to glaucoma.

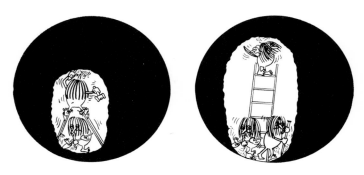

Fig. 2-17. Asynchronous upward and downward extension of optic cup orifice, which frequently occurs with glaucoma.

horizontal and vertical C/D ratios. One of the unfortunate problems with restricting evaluations of the optic nerve head to this method is the tendency of most observers, especially when using the direct ophthalmoscope, to judge the diameter of the cup on the basis of color rather than shape. This leads to erroneously small estimates of the glaucomatous cup's size because changes in shape precede changes in color. Furthermore, color alone is not a good guide for evaluating the progress of glaucoma, not because pallor is absent, but because its occurrence and location are sporadic, and because it is the loss of nerve tissue which is responsible for the visual dysfunction that occurs in the glaucomatous patient.

Gonioscopic Appearance

Basically, the question regarding all glaucomatous patients is "what is the appearance of the anterior chamber angle?" Because this area is hidden from view by the translucent limbus, it must be viewed by breaking up the total internal reflection of rays emanating from this area. A number of gonioscopic corneal contact lenses and techniques are

DISC DIAMETER ARBITRARILY SET
AT 1.00, THEN CUP DIAMETER IS
.3 OF THAT

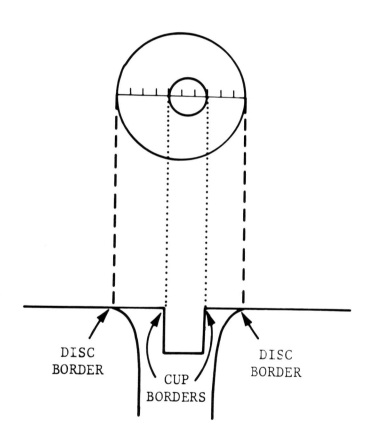

Fig. 2-18.   Estimation of the cup/disc ratio.

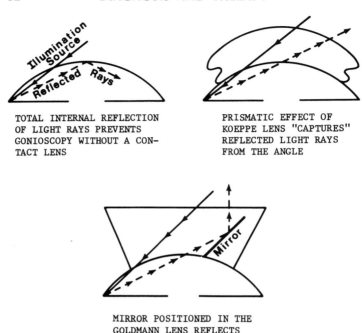

TOTAL INTERNAL REFLECTION
OF LIGHT RAYS PREVENTS
GONIOSCOPY WITHOUT A CON-
TACT LENS

PRISMATIC EFFECT OF
KOEPPE LENS "CAPTURES"
REFLECTED LIGHT RAYS
FROM THE ANGLE

MIRROR POSITIONED IN THE
GOLDMANN LENS REFLECTS
LIGHT RAYS EMERGING FROM
THE ANGLE

Fig. 2-19.   Appearance of the light rays from the angle and gonioscopic lenses and their effect.

available, each with its own advantages and disadvantages as compared to the others (Fig. 2–19).

The Koeppe prismatic lens, used with a ceiling-suspended microscope and a Barkan or a fiberoptics light, requires that the patient be supine. After topically anesthetizing the eye, the lens is applied and sterile water placed uniformly under it. The prismatic effect of this lens "captures" the internally reflected rays, and thereby provides a clear view of the angle. However, the magnification is not as good as that obtained with the following lenses.

The Goldmann, Allen-Thorpe, and Zeiss lenses are used at the slit lamp, the first two with methylcellulose under them and the latter with only tear film. All these lenses have mirrors in them that are set at the proper inclination to reflect rays coming from the angle. They are satisfactory for quick examination of the patient without requiring additional equipment or space for the patient to recline. These devices are particularly suited to opening a narrowed angle by applying direct pressure on the cornea. By so doing, an angle that is appositionally closed can be differentiated from one with apparent synechiae.

Whatever the instruments used, the accurate recognition of details in the chamber angle is the important matter. Anatom-

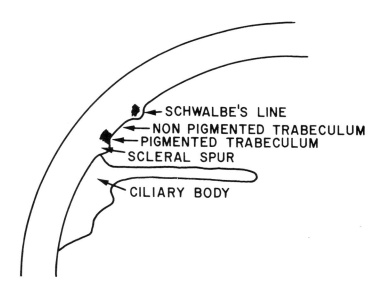

Fig. 2-20. Cross-sectional view of the anterior chamber angle.

ically, from anterior to posterior, the following structures and details must be sought (Fig. 2–20).

1. Schwalbe's line
2. trabeculum
   a. nonpigmented
   b. pigmented
3. scleral spur
4. ciliary body
5. estimation of the width of the angle between cornea and iris (its apex being the ciliary body.)

Each of these present special problems in visualization under various circumstances. Schwalbe's line is the termination of Descemet's membrane peripherally. Its appearance varies from a subtle, relatively grey interdigitation of the cornea and sclera to frank pigmentation resembling "the ring around a bathtub."

The trabeculum initially is not pigmented in the young eye. Gradually, pigment accumulates on its posterior extent, below before above, and faster in brown than in blue iris eyes. It is not uncommon to see no or very little pigmentation of the trabeculum in early open-angle glaucoma patients.

The scleral spur is the site of insertion of the ciliary body; it is white. The ciliary body stands out just behind it as grey or brown, being lighter in eyes with blue irides than in those with darker irides. These two angle structures offer little trouble in identification except in a patient with traumatic damage to that area (e.g., severe blow with traumatic cyclodialysis or angle recession). In these conditions, either the whiteness of the spur extends far posteriorly before the ciliary body is identified (traumatic cyclodialysis), or the spur is seen followed posteriorly by a tag of darker ciliary body followed by the stark whiteness of the scleral wall, or the ciliary body appears to be especially broad (angle recession). To determine the existence of subtle abnormalities in the angle, bilateral gonioscopy is valuable, allowing rapid back-and-forth comparison of symmetry, and this is most easily done with Koeppe lenses.

The presence of iris processes should be noted with regard to their location and density. They originate from the iris stroma, and in normal eyes, these are relatively sparse, inserting at the level of scleral spur. In many cases of primary open-angle glaucoma and pigmentary dispersion syndrome with glaucoma, these processes are more abundant and insert in great numbers anterior to their usual position. Some believe that the latter picture may indicate the presence of an underlying trabecular abnormality. **1992032**

The estimation of angle width is the most subjective of these five determinations. Normally, a wide, open angle will measure about 45 degrees. Angles less than 20 degrees are considered narrow. Estimating the likelihood of whether the angle is "not occludable," "possibly occludable," or "probably occludable" by a dilated and bunched up iris is important in every patient with a narrow angle. Unfortunately, this is best learned by the experience of examining many angles under a variety of circumstances, including mydriatic or dark provocation. In some cases the angle is narrowed but the anterior chamber is deep, giving the appearance of a plateau iris, an important differential diagnostic sign.

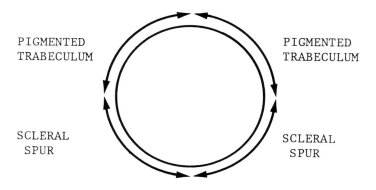

Fig. 2-21. Chart notation for recording the results of gonioscopy of the angle circumference.

While examining the angle for the location of normal tissues, inspection for cysts, tumors, foreign bodies, debris, neovascularization, membranes, synechiae, and inflammatory products is most important. To accurately document the position of each structure, a picture should be drawn using a clock-face geographic orientation (Fig. 2–21).

Provocative Tests

For open-angle glaucoma, the pilocarpine provocative test, the steroid provocative test, the PTC taste-test, and the water-drinking test have been utilized.

The pilocarpine provocative test can be used in one (preferably) or both eyes of a primary open-angle glaucoma suspect. One per cent pilocarpine is applied topically four times per day for one week. An intraocular pressure fall of 8 mm Hg or more is considered positive.

According to Becker, steroid responders can be broken down into nn, ng, and gg categories; these are genetic symbols established on the basis of the individual's response to steroids. The distribution in the population of these genotypes is about 63%, 33%, and 4% respectively. Typically, nn patients show no response to the application of topical steroids (six weeks of betamethasone q.i.d.); ng patients develop an intraocular pressure greater or equal to 20 mm Hg; and gg patients exceed 31 mm Hg. Increased intraocular pressure seems to correlate with a decrease in outflow facility. Patients with gg genotypes are supposedly prone to glaucoma. Other investigators have repeated this work. Although their statistics with regard to the amount of steroid-induced pressure rise vary, clearly different people do respond to steroids in different ways and do fall into three basic categories.

The PTC (phenylthiocarbamide) taste test has some limited value because a higher percentage of glaucomatous patients are nontasters (approximately 70%) than nonglaucomatous patients (approximately 30%). Since PTC tasting is genetically determined, this adds weight to the classification of steroid responders as a reflection of genetic determination.

Over the years, the water drinking test has seemed to be the most popular provocative test. A fasting patient is asked to drink one quart of water in five minutes. An increase of intraocular pressure of 8 mm Hg in 45 minutes, with pressures being taken at 10-minute intervals, is considered positive. Approximately 30% of glaucoma patients exhibit this response, which leaves a sizeable glaucomatous population undetected. In addition, some nonglaucomatous patients also respond positively. Combining this test with tonography does not seem to increase its usefulness.

In essence then, there is no absolutely confirmatory provocative test for open-angle glaucoma. The usefulness of these tests in diagnosis is limited, and they are used less frequently as quantitative perimetry and disc analysis become more common.

Facility of Outflow Measurement

Outflow facility (C value) is a measure of the ability of aqueous to leave the eye in a given period of time; it is expressed in units of μL/min/Hg. Decreased facility has many interpretations. Although there does appear to be a lower limit for normals at approximately .10, as an isolated finding the C value is even less reliable than pressure measurement. This is true because the outflow measurements of both normal individuals and glaucomatous patients fall within a broad range, with much cross-over between them. On the other hand, as many as 97.5% of normal persons may have outflow facilities greater than .17, but the exact percentage is not consistent. The reason for this apparent discrepancy in diagnostic value is that a reduced outflow is probably only one of the several factors necessary to produce a glaucomatous eye ("nerve head damageability" being another as yet unmeasured one).

Outflow is determined by placing a Schiøtz tonometer on the eye for four minutes and electronically recording the pressure during the time period. The weight of the tonometer forces additional aqueous out of the eye over and above the normal amount thereby reducing the intraocular pressure. The coefficient of outflow (C) is then calculated by using the equation:

$$C = \frac{\Delta V/T}{(P_{Tav} - P_0)}$$

ΔV = Change in intraocular volume due to the tonometer indentation and its weight on the eye

P_{Tav} = average intraocular pressure calculated with the addition of the tonometer weight on the eye

P_0 = initial intraocular pressure at zero (0) time calculated without the addition of the tonometer weight on the eye

T = time

Unfortunately, ΔV must be determined indirectly as is done in regular Schiøtz tonometry, so that the outflow facility is also indirectly measured. This is another reason why tonography is not an entirely helpful tool.

Nevertheless, the clinical computation process ignores these problems and simplifies it more by providing a nomogram that has been prepared from the basic equation (Tables 2–10, 2–11, 2–12). To use it, the scale reading at the beginning of the tracing is subtracted from that obtained four minutes later (Fig. 2–22). Using the nomogram particular to the tonometer weight that was employed, the column is identified that is headed by the value of the difference in readings that was just determined (ΔR). The appropriate row to be used on the nomogram is found by noting the initial reading at the start of the tracing (R_0). Then by sighting the junction of the row and column, one finally arrives at the C value.

Hidden in the measurement of C is another factor that makes the total facility of outflow falsely high, so that this parameter is called "pseudofacility." On the average, it accounts for .06 μL/min/Hg, and represents the decrease in aqueous production that occurs in response to the weight of the tonometer on the eye. This value must be subtracted from C to determine the "true" outflow facility.

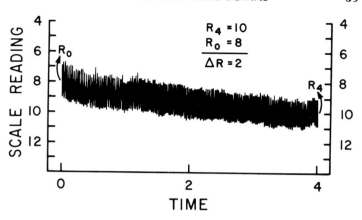

Fig. 2-22. Determination of change in tonographic reading from initial and final readings.

The flow rate of aqueous (F) can be determined by the following equation:

$$F = C (P_0 - P_e)$$

C = coefficient of outflow
P_0 = initial intraocular pressure at zero (0) time calculated without the addition of the tonometer weight on the eye
P_e = episcleral venous pressure

Eight is the average episcleral venous pressure in millimeters of mercury. In addition, the P_0/C can be calculated. This ratio is apparently more sensitive than C alone. As many as 97.5% of normal eyes do not exceed a P_0/C of 100, while the overlap with glaucomatous eyes is even less than for C. Unfortunately, both F and P_0/C are also indirect measurements, which suffer from the inherent errors of tonography that have already been described.

Table 2-10. Nomogram for Coefficient of Outflow (C) From Tonograms Using the 5.5-gm Weight (µL/min/mm Hg).

INITIAL READING		5.5 gm wt ΔR (change in scale reading)										
P_0	R	0	.50	1.00	1.50	2.00	2.50	3.00	3.50	4.00	4.50	5.00
24	3.00	0	.04	.09	.14	.20	.27	.35	.44	.54	.65	.78
23	3.25	0	.04	.09	.14	.20	.26	.33	.42	.51	.62	.74
22	3.50	0	.04	.08	.13	.19	.25	.32	.40	.49	.59	.70
22	3.75	0	.04	.08	.13	.19	.25	.31	.38	.47	.56	.66
21	4.00	0	.04	.08	.13	.18	.24	.30	.37	.45	.54	.63
20	4.25	0	.04	.08	.13	.18	.24	.30	.36	.43	.52	.60
19	4.50	0	.04	.08	.12	.17	.23	.29	.35	.42	.50	.58
18	4.75	0	.04	.08	.12	.17	.23	.28	.34	.41	.48	.56
17	5.00	0	.04	.08	.12	.17	.22	.27	.33	.40	.47	.54
17	5.25	0	.04	.08	.12	.17	.22	.27	.33	.39	.46	.53

16	5.50	0	.04	.08	.12	.16	.21	.26	.32	.38	.45	.52
15	5.75	0	.04	.08	.12	.16	.21	.26	.32	.38	.44	.50
15	6.00	0	.03	.07	.11	.15	.20	.25	.31	.37	.43	.49
14	6.25	0	.03	.07	.11	.15	.20	.25	.31	.37	.43	.49
13	6.50	0	.03	.07	.11	.15	.20	.25	.30	.36	.42	.48
13	6.75	0	.03	.07	.11	.15	.20	.24	.30	.36	.41	.47
12	7.00	0	.03	.07	.11	.15	.20	.24	.29	.35	.40	.46
11	7.50	0	.03	.07	.11	.15	.19	.24	.29	.34	.39	.45
10	8.00	0	.03	.07	.11	.15	.19	.24	.29	.34	.39	.45
9	8.50	0	.03	.07	.11	.15	.19	.23	.28	.33	.39	
9	9.00	0	.03	.07	.11	.15	.19	.23	.28	.33		
8	9.50	0	.03	.07	.11	.15	.19	.23	.28			
7	10.00	0	.03	.07	.11	.15	.19	.23				
6	11.00	0	.03	.07	.11	.15						

(From Ballintine, E. J.: Tonographic technique. Trans. Am. Acad. Ophthalmol. Otolaryngol. 65:136–144, 1961.)

Table 2-11. Nomogram for Coefficient of Outflow (C) From Tonograms Using the 7.5-gm Weight (μL/min/mm Hg).

INITIAL READING		7.5 gm-wt ΔR (change in scale reading)										
P_0	R	0	.50	1.00	1.50	2.00	2.50	3.00	3.50	4.00	4.50	5.00
36	3.00	0	.03	.07	.12	.17	.23	.31	.40	.50	.62	.76
34	3.25	0	.03	.07	.12	.17	.22	.29	.37	.46	.57	.69
33	3.50	0	.03	.07	.11	.16	.21	.28	.35	.43	.53	.63
32	3.75	0	.03	.07	.11	.16	.21	.26	.33	.41	.49	.59
30	4.00	0	.03	.06	.10	.15	.20	.25	.32	.39	.46	.55
29	4.25	0	.03	.06	.10	.15	.19	.25	.30	.37	.44	.52
28	4.50	0	.03	.06	.10	.14	.18	.24	.29	.35	.42	.50
27	4.75	0	.03	.06	.10	.14	.18	.23	.28	.34	.40	.47
26	5.00	0	.03	.06	.10	.13	.17	.22	.27	.33	.39	.45
25	5.25	0	.03	.06	.10	.13	.17	.22	.27	.32	.38	.43

24	5.50	0	.03	.06	.09	.13	.16	.21	.26	.31	.37	.42
23	5.75	0	.03	.06	.09	.13	.16	.21	.26	.31	.36	.41
22	6.00	0	.03	.06	.09	.12	.16	.20	.25	.30	.35	.40
21	6.25	0	.03	.06	.09	.12	.16	.20	.25	.29	.34	.39
20	6.50	0	.03	.05	.09	.12	.15	.19	.24	.28	.33	.38
19	6.75	0	.03	.05	.09	.12	.15	.19	.24	.28	.33	.38
18	7.00	0	.03	.05	.08	.12	.15	.19	.23	.27	.32	.37
17	7.50	0	.03	.05	.08	.12	.15	.19	.23	.27	.31	.36
16	8.00	0	.03	.05	.08	.11	.15	.18	.22	.26	.30	.35
14	8.50	0	.03	.05	.08	.11	.15	.18	.22	.26	.30	
13	9.00	0	.03	.05	.08	.11	.15	.18	.22	.25		
12	9.50	0	.03	.05	.08	.11	.15	.18	.22			
11	10.00	0	.03	.05	.08	.11	.14	.18				
10	11.00	0	.03	.05	.08	.11	.14					

(From Ballintine, E. J.: Tonographic technique. Trans. Am. Acad. Ophthalmol. Otolaryngol. 65:136–144, 1961.)

Table 2-12. Nomogram for Coefficient of Outflow (C) From Tonograms Using the 10.0-gm Weight (μL/min/mm Hg).

INITIAL READING		10.0 gm wt ΔR (change in scale reading)										
P_o	R	0	.50	1.00	1.50	2.00	2.50	3.00	3.50	4.00	4.50	5.00
51	3.00	0	.03	.06	.10	.15	.21	.29	.38	.49		
49	3.25	0	.03	.06	.10	.14	.20	.27	.35	.44		
47	3.50	0	.03	.06	.09	.13	.19	.25	.32	.40	.50	
45	3.75	0	.03	.06	.09	.13	.18	.23	.30	.37	.46	
43	4.00	0	.02	.05	.08	.12	.17	.22	.28	.35	.43	.52
42	4.25	0	.02	.05	.08	.12	.17	.21	.26	.33	.40	.48
40	4.50	0	.02	.05	.07	.11	.16	.20	.25	.31	.38	.44
38	4.75	0	.02	.05	.07	.11	.16	.20	.24	.29	.36	.42
37	5.00	0	.02	.05	.07	.10	.15	.19	.23	.28	.34	.40
36	5.25	0	.02	.05	.07	.10	.15	.19	.23	.27	.32	.38
34	5.50	0	.02	.05	.07	.10	.14	.18	.22	.26	.31	.36
33	5.75	0	.02	.05	.07	.10	.14	.18	.22	.25	.30	.34

32	6.00	0	.02	.04	.07	.10	.13	.17	.21	.24	.29	.33
31	6.25	0	.02	.04	.07	.10	.13	.17	.21	.24	.28	.32
29	6.50	0	.02	.04	.07	.10	.13	.16	.20	.23	.27	.31
28	6.75	0	.02	.04	.07	.10	.13	.16	.20	.23	.27	.31
27	7.00	0	.02	.04	.07	.09	.12	.15	.19	.22	.26	.30
26	7.25	0	.02	.04	.07	.09	.12	.15	.19	.22	.26	.30
25	7.50	0	.02	.04	.07	.09	.12	.15	.18	.21	.25	.29
24	7.75	0	.02	.04	.07	.09	.12	.15	.18	.21	.25	.29
23	8.00	0	.02	.04	.06	.09	.12	.14	.18	.21	.24	.28
21	8.50	0	.02	.04	.06	.09	.11	.14	.18	.20	.23	.27
20	9.00	0	.02	.04	.06	.09	.11	.14	.17	.20	.23	.26
18	9.50	0	.02	.04	.06	.09	.11	.14	.17	.20	.23	.26
16	10.00	0	.02	.04	.06	.09	.11	.14	.17	.19·	.22	.26
14	11.00	0	.02	.04	.06	.09	.11	.14	.17	.19	.22	.25

(From Ballintine, E. J.: Tonographic technique. Trans. Am. Acad. Ophthalmol. Otolaryngol. 65:136–144, 1961.)

45

GENERAL DIFFERENCES BETWEEN PRIMARY AND SECONDARY OPEN-ANGLE GLAUCOMA

Both types of open-angle glaucoma are diagnosed in the same way except for one major difference: in secondary open-angle glaucoma, the obstruction to outflow frequently can be identified. To do so, however, sometimes requires a high level of investigation, suspicion, and acumen. This will be discussed later in detail.

As previously mentioned, pressure readings alone are not sufficient for diagnosis of primary open-angle glaucoma. The presence of a characteristic scotoma is the sine qua non of this disease. If no visual field defects are found, however, then only the evaluation of the optic cup is available on which to base the diagnosis. Fortunately, present methods of optic disc analysis have permitted diagnosticians to attain a higher degree of confidence in the appearance of the cup than ever before. In fact, it is entirely possible to suspect glaucomatous damage to an optic nerve head and not find visual field loss with even the most thorough testing, so that careful and accurate disc examination may well become *the* issue on which the ultimate management decision is finally based.

TREATMENT OF PRIMARY OPEN-ANGLE GLAUCOMA

Medical Management

Three kinds of drugs are clinically available for medical treatment: parasympathetic stimulators, sympathetic stimulators, and carbonic anhydrase inhibitors (Tables 2–13, 2–14).

The first category (parasympathetics) can be subdivided into (1) parasympathomimetics, such as pilocarpine and carbachol, which act directly on the parasympathetic end plates, and (2) cholinesterase inhibitors, such as echothiophate and demecarium bromide, which are longer-acting and promote the retention of acetylcholine. All of these medications

Table 2-13. Antiglaucomatous Eye Drops (%).

	Pilocarpine (q.i.d.)	Carbachol (t.i.d.)	Echothiophate (b.i.d.)	Demecarium bromide (b.i.d.)	Free base epinephrine (once daily or b.i.d.)
Minimal dose	.5	.75	.03	—	.25
Ordinary dose range	1 2 3 4	1.50 2.25 3.00	.06 .125 .250	.125 .250	.50 1.00
High dose	6 8 10				2.00

Table 2-14. Antiglaucomatous Pills.

Generic name	Acetazolamide	Methazolamide	Ethoxzolamide	Dichlorphenamide
Brand name	Diamox, Hydrazol	Neptazane	Ethamide, Cardrase	Daranide, Oratrol
Manufacturer's recommended dose	125 mg b.i.d. to 250 mg q.i.d.	50 mg b.i.d. to 100 mg t.i.d.	125 mg b.i.d. to 125 mg q.i.d.	25 mg daily to 50 mg t.i.d.

function by increasing the true facility of outflow, possibly by causing the longitudinal ciliary muscle to contract, which in turn may open the trabecular pores more widely. In addition, pilocarpine appears to increase the pseudofacility, which enhances the reduction of vascular filtration of aqueous as the intraocular pressure increases during its diurnal cycle.

The second category (sympathetics) is represented by epinephrine. Its mode of action appears to be primarily related to inflow reduction (beta effect) and pseudofacility reduction (alpha effect). Both of these effects have been reported to be more dramatic in younger people than in older people.

The third category of drugs (carbonic anhydrase inhibitors) consists of acetazolamide, methazolamide, ethoxzolamide and dichlorphenamide, which work by interfering with the active secretion of aqueous by the ciliary body (a reduction of more than 40% in most glaucomatous eyes).

With regard to the appropriate dose of these medications, the following regimens might be used as standards from which individual variations can be made.

Phakic patients should usually be started on pilocarpine 1% as soon as it is decided that treatment is necessary. Progression to pilocarpine 2% would be the next step, followed by the addition of epinephrine ½%. After this the pilocarpine strength might be raised to 4% followed by an increase of epinephrine to 1%. For many people one of these steps is all that is needed to control the pressure, at least initially.

Aphakic patients might be started on .06% echothiophate followed by increases in dosage to .125% and then .25%. If this is still insufficient, the use of epinephrine free base, .25% or .5% is warranted. However, because of the incidence of maculopathy in aphakic patients receiving epinephrine, these patients must be watched closely and the medicine discontinued if macular edema appears.

If dosages of topical medications have been brought up to the ordinary maximum and the pressure is still unacceptable, the use of carbonic anhydrase inhibitors is warranted. For example, acetazolamide may be started in a dose of 125 mg b.i.d. and finally increased to 250 mg q.i.d. if necessary. Although it has been suggested that these drugs are less likely to cause complications, recent evidence has begun to refute this claim. Of special concern are the side effects of kidney stone formation and metabolic acidosis, the latter being particulary hazardous in uncontrolled diabetics. A more substantial advantage of switching therapy among the different products is the relief of nausea, numbness, or tingling, which seem to vary in degree depending on the specific drug used. Unfortunately, these symptoms make it impossible for some people to take any carbonic anhydrase inhibitor.

Topical medications may also present some special problems. For example, if carbachol (a slightly more potent drug) is used to replace pilocarpine, as is sometimes desirable in patients whose pressure is hard to control, it may cause intolerable conjunctival irritation. A satisfactory alternative might be the use of sustained-release devices. Inserts containing medication are placed in the conjunctival cul de sac weekly and can be a great convenience if they are sufficiently effective and stay in position.

The physician must pay careful attention to the percentage of free base and anion of epinephrine preparations, because these factors influence the degree of ocular discomfort (bitartrate being the worst) and the potency of the drug (Table 2–15).

If all other treatment fails, the use of echothiophate on a trial basis in phakic patients is warranted, especially in one eye. Unfortunately, this drug has the undesirable side effect of causing cataract or iris cyst formation in susceptible individuals.

The short-term evaluation of response to these medications is usually based on intraocular pressure measurements. In patients whose intraocular tension is not dangerously high, using a drop in only one eye helps to make a rapid determination of patient response to therapy. By so doing, the normal diurnal fluctuations in pressure (which are particularly

Table 2-15. Epinephrine Products.

Trade Name	Anion	Percent Free Base in a 1% Solution	Solution Dose Range (%)
Epifrin, Glaucon	Hydrochloride	1.00	.25 to 2.00
Epinal, Eppy	Borate	1.00	.25 to 1.00
Epitrate, Mytrate, E1	Bitartrate	.55	1.00 to 2.00

large in glaucoma) can be seen in the other eye, and the effects of medication can be compared with these variations. When this is not done, a pressure measurement taken at the low ebb of the diurnal curve may be inadvertently confused with successful therapy. Finding an improved coefficient of outflow while on medication can be a useful additional sign.

If a person on treatment does *not* show visual field loss, it seems wise to prescribe the least amount of medication(s) that lowers the pressure reading to the lower twenties. There is no reason to exhaust one's medication reserves to combat visual field loss, which might never occur. If field loss does occur eventually, then a medical regimen is still available for therapy before surgical intervention becomes necessary. In most patients with visual field loss, lowering the intraocular pressure below 20 mm Hg is essential to prevent progression of the disease.

Surgical Decisions

The indications for surgical intervention vary widely among ophthalmologists, and range from "almost never" to "not infrequently." The major reasons responsible for the hesitation to perform surgery are the following:

1. Increased rate of cataract formation in eyes operated on for glaucoma.
2. Increased risk of endophthalmitis.
3. The possibility of surgical failure, which varies, in part, according to the technique and the experience of surgeon.
4. Reports of complete loss of visual field or development of markedly less acute central vision after operation on some advanced glaucomatous eyes (not well documented).
5. The risk of surgical complications in any operative procedure (e.g., flat anterior chamber leading to anterior synechia formation, and development of angle-closure glaucoma).

An approach to this dilemma might be the adoption of the following rules:

1. Operate only on an eye that has continued to lose visual field despite "maximal medication."
2. Never operate on an eye without at *least* definite reproducible visual field loss, no matter what the patient's age, unless there is persistent high pressure or resultant pain, corneal edema, and loss of visual acuity.

The question of what constitutes maximal medication varies from patient to patient. Obviously, pilocarpine 4% q.i.d., epinephrine 1% b.i.d., and acetazolamide 250 mg q.i.d. is very strong medication but it is not necessarily maximal. Switching to carbachol or echothiophate, changing brands of epinephrine or carbonic anhydrase inhibitors should all be tried to be sure of identifying which medications are most effective for a particular patient. A young person who experiences blurring from pilocarpine may find that clipping on minus lenses or using epinephrine instead is more comfortable. If it is not, if the patient has intolerable side effects from carbonic anhydrase inhibitors, or if the ophthalmologist does not wish to subject him to the long-term use of these drugs, then it may be necessary to operate if there is reproducible glaucomatous field loss. On the other hand, a 75-year-old person with some medication intolerance and moderate field loss may never be a candidate for surgical intervention. Before an operation is performed, however, even a phakic patient might be given a trial regimen of echothiophate, despite the higher incidence of cataract formation in these instances. This can be justified on the basis of the significant percentage of surgical failures and complications that still occur. An aphakic person is a better candidate for this drug, but it may not lower the intraocular pressure sufficiently. This patient, even though aphakic, may respond better to pilocarpine or carbachol.

Experimentation within this framework is warranted before subjecting any patient to surgery. This is not to say that surgical operation for open-angle glaucoma should be avoided at all costs. It should be reserved for those people with well observed, advanced, or advancing visual field loss.

Operative Procedures

In a phakic patient, the choice of filtering procedures are:

1. anterior lip sclerectomy
2. posterior lip sclerectomy
3. thermosclerotomy
4. trephination
5. trabeculectomy
6. iridencleisis

In an aphakic patient, surgical cyclodialysis might be considered instead of one of the foregoing procedures.

Table 2-16. Differences Among Filtering Procedures.

Type of Procedure	Tissue Excised	Tissue Incised
Anterior lip sclerectomy	Anterior limbus (punch)	Posterior limbus (knife)
Posterior lip sclerectomy	Posterior limbus (punch)	Anterior limbus (knife)
Thermosclerotomy	None	Posterior limbus (knife and cautery)
Trephination	Full-thickness posterior limbus and sclera (trephine)	None
Trabeculectomy	Partial-thickness limbus and sclera under the flap (knife, trephine or scissors)	Partial-thickness limbus and scleral flap (knife)
Iridencleisis	None (iris is incarcerated in wound)	Posterior limbus (knife)

Each procedure calls for a somewhat different approach to producing external fistulization (Table 2–16), and each has its own particular advantages and disadvantages. Some are technically more difficult than others. Some are more disfiguring, some are more likely to close postoperatively, and some endanger the lens more than others. Presently, the trabeculectomy seems most promising with regard to success of filtration and minimization of complications. However, it does not always lower the intraocular pressure to the very low levels obtained with other successful procedures.

Recent evidence that lens extraction alone "cures" glaucoma in over 50% of people makes it the operation of choice in a glaucoma patient with an advanced senile cataract. This approach has greatly reduced the use of the combined lens extraction-filtering procedure. However, when the latter approach is desired, the trabeculectomy and lens extraction work exceedingly well together.

DIAGNOSIS AND TREATMENT OF SECONDARY OPEN-ANGLE GLAUCOMA

Basically, the differences in diagnosis and treatment of secondary open-angle glaucoma as compared to primary open-angle glaucoma come from the discovery of the primary disease and the limitations it imposes.

Inflammatory Causes

Anterior Uveitis. Resistance to outflow increases because inflammatory products are present in or on the meshwork. Treatment must be aimed at counteracting the inflammation by the use of steroids, despite the fact that steroids will cause an additional increase in pressure in some patients (although some steroids are less likely than others to raise the ocular tension). Hopefully, the inflammation will subside rapidly and the eye will be capable of withstanding a short-term elevation in pressure. Quite probably, the tension can be controlled with epinephrine and carbonic anhydrase inhibitors. After the acute inflammation has been controlled, treatment can proceed as in primary open-angle glaucoma if necessary. Frequently, however, the pressure will become normal without any medication.

Some of these cases are actually part of the syndrome called Fuchs heterochromic iridocyclitis. There is a low grade cyclitis with fine keratic precipitates which seems to produce no synechiae. It is usually unilateral and associated with lightening of the iris color. Cataract frequently forms as a complication. Unfortunately, the elevation of pressure associated with this disease does not ordinarily relent as the inflammation clears with therapy.

Reaction to Lens Cortex. Inflammation secondary to sensitivity to lens material can occur in a variety of forms. Phacolytic glaucoma and phacoanaphylactic uveitis are two such types. Phacolytic glaucoma is due to macrophagic blockage of the trabeculum that occurs in response to leakage of protein through the capsule of mature or hypermature lenses. Phacoanaphylactic glaucoma occurs because of giant and epithelioid cell obstruction to outflow. These cells enter the anterior chamber subsequent to a previous sensitization to lens material, as when there has been an extracapsular extraction. This reaction may even occur in the "other" originally normal eye. In both kinds of glaucoma, lens extraction should be performed after medical reduction of intraocular pressure. In cases of phacoanaphylactic reaction, it may be necessary to operate on the inciting eye to remove retained lens fragments that were left behind during the initial surgery.

Alphachymotrypsin. This glaucoma is caused by blockage of the trabecular meshwork with lysed zonular material after using this enzyme to facilitate cataract extraction. The pressure elevation is usually controllable with carbonic anhydrase inhibitors; it gradually subsides within a matter of days, even without therapy, as the zonules make their way through the outflow channels.

Glaucomatocyclitic Crisis. A syndrome of unilateral, recurrent, severe elevations of pressure that may last a few hours to weeks; the symptoms include mild discomfort, blurring of vision, mild anterior chamber inflammation, and even keratic precipitates. Cycloplegia combined with carbonic anhydrase inhibitors is usually successful in overcoming the attacks. Although it was originally believed that these eyes were completely normal during the periods of remission, recent data suggest that they do show many of the signs of primary open-angle glaucoma.

Traumatic Causes

Angle Contusion. A severe blow to the eye may sooner or later cause an increase in intraocular pressure. Studies support the idea that a tear of the ciliary body (angle recession) or traumatic cyclodialysis cannot be correlated with the long-term effect on intraocular pressure. In a recent ten-year follow up on such eyes, only 9% had developed glaucoma, although it took a full ten years for this to occur in one case. Thus, patients with gonioscopic evidence of trauma to the angle require an annual eye examination at the minimum.

Supposedly, the damage sustained by the trabecular meshwork is the crucial factor. The degree of damage is difficult to evaluate clinically. However, almost all cases of angle contusion glaucoma have angle recessions of 180 degrees or more, which suggests that a severe injury is the basis for the rise in pressure. When glaucoma does occur in an eye in which the longitudinal muscle of the ciliary body has been interrupted, pilocarpine may not be fully effective, since its mode of action seems to depend in part on the pull of this muscle on the trabeculum. In these cases epinephrine may be more useful. Except for this problem, the treatment of postcontusion glaucomatous eyes is similar to that for primary open-angle glaucoma.

Lens Dislocation. Posterior dislocation sometimes increases the intraocular pressure. This may be due to a coincident pupillary block by the vitreous, angle recession, anterior synechia formation, or another cause that cannot be found. Nevertheless, the lens should not be removed unless the glaucoma is phacolytic in origin and the eye shows an inflammatory reaction in the anterior chamber. Otherwise, treatment should proceed along standard lines for primary open-angle glaucoma.

Anterior lens dislocation into the anterior chamber is an indication for lens extraction to prevent damage to the cornea, pupillary block, or direct obstruction of the angle (see angle-closure glaucoma).

Neovascular-Hemorrhagic Causes

Incipient Angle Neovascularization. This term is used to refer to early neovascular glaucoma associated with rubeosis iridis but occurring before advanced neovascularization of the angle is present. It is caused most commonly by diabetic retinopathy (33%) and central retinal vein occlusion (28%), although it is not often part of these diseases. Initially, increased intraocular pressure may be found without obvious angle obstruction, though a few new vessels may be seen coursing over an open angle. In advanced stages, one can gonioscopically identify a closed angle from a neovascular *membrane* covering the trabeculum. Some other conditions in which neovascular glaucoma occurs are chronic uveitis, carotid disease, retinal detachment, and intraocular tumor.

Traditionally, these open-angle eyes are medically treated like primary open-angle glaucoma. It seems prudent to consider filtering surgery earlier than would ordinarily be the case, because many eyes with neovascular glaucoma become blind when treated only with medication. Unfortunately, when the physician is finally forced to operate, the risk of bleeding from newly formed vessels frequently precludes surgical intervention, and the failure rate is inordinately high. To avoid this situation, a filtering procedure on one eye of such a patient may be indicated at an early stage in his glaucoma. For many of these patients, however, cyclo-cryothermy to reduce aqueous formation is the only plausible treatment, although not an especially effective one. Recent trials of pan-retinal photocoagulation for this disease appear promising but are not conclusive as yet.

Anterior Chamber Hemorrhage. Blood in the anterior chamber will raise the intraocular pressure if hemolyzed red blood cells and hemoglobin-laden macrophages retard outflow or if whole erythrocytes or their ghost cells sufficiently obstruct the trabeculum. The minimum hyphema level necessary for this is unclear, but would seem to be at least one-half of the anterior chamber. Attempts at maintaining normal intraocular pressure with carbonic anhydrase inhibitors may be successful. However, after a few days of intractable elevated intraocular pressure, the anterior chamber should be opened and emptied; otherwise, the danger of blood staining of the cornea and trabecular hemosiderosis with permanent damage become real possibilities. Even without increased pressure, a total hyphema should be removed if it shows no signs of resolving after five days.

Syndrome-Related Causes

Pigmentary Dispersion. This syndrome is characterized by a heavy accumulation of pigment on the trabecular surface, deposits of pigment on the corneal endothelium (Krukenberg spindle, if it is relatively linear), a loss of iris pigment posteriorly in a concentric midperipheral zone, and relatively dense iris processes that insert above the scleral spur. The syndome occurs most often in young adult myopic males. Pressure elevation may be intermittent or variable, which is supposedly related to the amount of pigment that can be discharged through the trabecular apparatus at one time. On the other hand, many people have heavy accumulations of anterior and even posterior chamber pigment but never develop glaucoma, so that some doubt exists regarding the mechanism involved. Treatment is the same as primary open-angle glaucoma, of which this seems to be a variant.

(Pseudo) Exfoliation. In this syndrome, an amorphous dandruff-like material is deposited, among other places, anteriorly on the lens capsule surface and rubs pigment off the posterior iris, especially near the pupil. The origin of this material may be from zonules, lens, iris or ciliary body but clinically resembles true exfoliation of the lens capsule, hence the term (pseudo) exfoliation. The loosened iris pigment accumulates in heavy amounts on the trabecular meshwork, which may cause the increase of intraocular pressure. Furthermore, the (pseudo) exfoliated material has been found to clog the trabecular interspaces. Because such (pseudo) exfoliation frequently occurs without glaucoma, the mechanism involved here is also in doubt. This disease should be treated as for primary open-angle glaucoma, although the incidence of early disc and visual field change is much higher in the (pseudo) exfoliation syndrome. Usually, the glaucoma is unilateral, but in most cases the fellow eye has a mildly increased intraocular pressure or decreased facility of outflow as well. This suggests that (pseudo) exfoliation syndrome may be just another form of primary open-angle glaucoma that is extremely asymmetric in presentation.

SUGGESTED READINGS

Armaly, M.F.: Selective perimetry for glaucomatous defects in ocular hypertension. Arch. Ophthalmol. 87:518-524, 1972. (Sets criteria for determining when nasal step, paracentral scotoma, and concentric isopter contraction are significant defects.)

———: Ocular pressure and visual fields. Arch. Ophthalmol. 81:25-40, 1969. (Four out of 10,000 normal patients developed glaucoma after 10 years follow up.)

———: The size and location of the normal blind spot. Arch. Ophthalmol. 81:192-201, 1969. (Retinal blur from a small pupil or a poor refraction can cause an enlargement of the blind spot.)

———: The heritable nature of dexamethasone-induced ocular hypertension. Arch. Ophthalmol. 75:32-35, 1966. (Three genetic patient categories of steroid-induced intraocular pressure elevation can be established on the basis of whether it rises < 6 mm Hg (P^lP^l), 6 to 15 mm Hg (P^lP^h), or ≥ 16 mm Hg (P^hP^h).

Barany, E. H.: A mathematical formulation of intraocular pressure as dependent on secretion, ultrafiltration, bulk outflow, and osmotic reabsorption of fluid. Invest. Ophthalmol. 2:584-590, 1963. (A detailed mathematical formulation of these components of aqueous dynamics.)

Barsam, P. C.: Comparison of the effect of pilocarpine and echothiophate on intraocular pressure and outflow facility. Am. J. Ophthalmol. 73:742-749, 1972. (In the 2% and .06% strength, respectively, these drugs lower intraocular pressure to a similar level, but echothiophate acts longer.)

Becker, B.: Intraocular pressure response to topical corticosteroids. Invest. Ophthalmol. 4:198-205, 1965. (There are three genetic populations of responders—nn, ng and gg—whose pressure after steroid provocation rises respectively to < 20 mm Hg, ≥ 20 mm Hg, or > 31 mm Hg.)

————: Tonometry, tonography and provocative tests in the management of the glaucomas. Trans. Am. Acad. Ophthalmol. Otolaryngol. 64:127-134, 1960. (Of known glaucomatous eyes, 28% demonstrate a rise of 8 mm Hg+ in intraocular pressure after ingestion of a liter of water, but 97% develop a P_0/C over 100.)

————: Use of methazolamide (Neptazane) in the therapy of glaucoma. Am. J. Ophthalmol. 49:1307-1311, 1960. (Methazolamide is not quite as effective as acetazolamide, but a lower dose of medication is needed and fewer side effects occur.)

Becker, B., and Morton, W. R.: Phenylthiourea taste testing and glaucoma. Arch. Ophthalmol. 72:323-327, 1964. (The percentage of nontasting in normal vs. glaucomatous patients is as follows: Caucasians 28%:53%, Negroes 17%:31%.)

Becker, S. C. : Unrecognized errors induced by present-day gonioprisms and a proposal for their elimination. Arch. Ophthalmol. 82:160-168, 1969. (The gonioscopic view can be improved by using a lens that is designed for the particular patient's corneal curvature and anterior chamber depth.)

Begg, I. S., Drance, S. M., and Sweeney, V.P.: Hemorrhage on the disc—A sign of acute ischaemic optic neuropathy in chronic simple glaucoma. Can. J. Ophthalmol. 5:321-330, 1970. (The later development of visual field defects can be correlated with the location of the previous hemorrhage.)

Bigger, J. F., and Becker, B.: Cataracts and primary open-angle glaucoma: The effect of uncomplicated cataract extraction on glaucoma control. Trans. Am. Acad. Ophthalmol. Otolaryngol. 75:260-272, 1971. (Of patients with glaucoma, 56% showed an improvement of intraocular pressure or decrease in need for medication one year later.)

Brais, P., and Drance, S. M.: The temporal field in chronic simple glaucoma. Arch. Ophthalmol. 88:518-522, 1972. (Temporal scotomas, such as radial nerve fiber bundle defects, and wedge-shaped defects, occur in some eyes with early glaucoma.)

Cairns, J. E.: Trabeculectomy. Preliminary report of a new method. Am. J. Ophthalmol. 66:673-679, 1968. (A description of the technique.)

deRoetth, A.: Clinical evaluation of tonography. Am. J. Ophthalmol. 59:169-179, 1965. (There is a wide overlap of the range of values for normal and glaucoma patients.)

Drance, S. M.: Medical management of early chronic open angle glaucoma. *In* Symposium on Glaucoma, 23rd, 1974: Transactions of the New Orleans Academy of Ophthalmology. pp. 68-80. St. Louis, C. V. Mosby Co., 1975. (Personal views on how to treat glaucoma.)

———: The early field defects in glaucoma. Invest. Ophthalmol. 8:84-91, 1969. (Uses static perimetry to prove the significance of small kinetic defects, such as paracentral scotomata, and to disprove the significance of baring of the blind spot in glaucoma.)

Drance, S. M., Sweeney, V. P., Morgan, R. W., and Feldman, F.: Studies of factors involved in the production of low tension glaucoma. Arch. Ophthalmol. 89:457-465, 1973. (Emphasizes the frequency of hemodynamic crises and vascular disease in these patients.)

Drance, S. M., and Vargas, E.: Trabeculectomy and thermosclerectomy: A comparison of two procedures. Can. J. Ophthalmol. 8:413-415, 1973. (Pressure control is the same but anterior chamber depth and lens clarity are better after trabeculectomy.)

Feibel, R. M., and Bigger, J. F.: Rubeosis iridis and neovascular glaucoma: Evaluation of cyclocryotherapy. Am. J. Ophthalmol. 74:862-867, 1972. (An approximate 50% success rate.)

Flocks, M., Littwin, C. S., and Zimmerman, L. E.: Phacolytic glaucoma. Arch. Ophthalmol. 54:37-45, 1955. (Macrophages engulf liquified lens cortex that has leaked through the capsule and thereby block the trabecular meshwork.)

Goldmann, H.: An analysis of some concepts concerning chronic simple glaucoma. Am. J. Ophthalmol. 80:409-416, 1975. (The height of the intraocular pressure needed to produce glaucomatous damage is not the same in all patients.)

Haas, J. S.: Surgical treatment of open-angle glaucoma. *In* Symposium on Glaucoma, 15th, 1966: Transactions of the New Orleans Academy of Ophthalmology. pp. 175-186. St. Louis, C. V. Mosby Co., 1967. (Operate when glaucomatous damage occurs despite medical therapy or when it is judged that damage would otherwise be unavoidable.)

Harbin, T. S., and Pollack, I. P.: Glaucoma in episcleritis. Arch. Ophthalmol. 93:948-950, 1975. (The cause of the increased pressure appears to be an adjacent trabeculitis.)

Harris, L. S., Galin, M. A., and Lerner, R.: The influence of low dose L-epinephrine on intraocular pressure. Ann. Ophthalmol. 2:253-257, 1970. (Although as little as .06% epinephrine may be effective in reducing intraocular pressure, strengths as high as 2% may be needed in some cases to achieve a useful hypotensive response.)

Henkind, P.: Angle vessels in normal eyes. Brit. J. Opthalmol. 48: 551-557, 1964. (There are three normal types of vessels in the angle: circular ciliary or radial iris from the major circle, and radial ciliary from the deep scleral plexus.)

Horven, I.: Exfoliation syndrome. Arch. Ophthalmol. 76:505-511, 1966. (Although prevalent in Scandinavians, this disease respects no national boundaries; it is much more severe than primary open-angle glaucoma and causes heavy pigmentation of the trabecular meshwork.)

Hoskins, H. D.: Neovascular glaucoma: Current concepts. Trans. Am. Acad. Ophthalmol. Otolaryngol. 78:330-333, 1974. (Diabetes, central retinal vein occlusion, iritis, carotid disease and trauma are the most common causes.)

————: Interpretive gonioscopy in glaucoma. Invest. Ophthalmol. 11:97-102, 1972. (Rotating an indirect gonioscopic lens toward a narrow angle permits fuller visibility of its depth; unless the slit beam from the cornea meets the one from the iris, the junction of these tissues is not in view.)

Howard, G. M., Hutchinson, B. T., and Frederick, A. R.: Hyphema resulting from blunt trauma. Trans. Am. Acad. Ophthalmol. Otolaryngol. 69:294-306, 1965. (The appearance of angle recession varies from disinsertion of the iris processes, through various degrees of tears in the ciliary body, to traumatic cyclodialysis.)

Iliff, C. E., and Haas, J. S.: Posterior lip sclerectomy. Am. J. Ophthalmol. 54:688-693, 1962. (A description of the technique.)

Jerndal, T., and Lundström, M.: Trabeculectomy combined with cataract extraction. Am. J. Ophthalmol. 81:227-231, 1976. (This procedure controlled the intraocular pressure in 82% of patients and the complications were minimal.)

Kass, M. A., Becker, B., and Kolker, A. E.: Glaucomatocyclitic crisis and primary open-angle glaucoma. Am. J. Ophthalmol. 75:668-673, 1973. (Both eyes in this supposedly unilateral and transient condition show signs of glaucoma even between attacks.)

Kaufman, H. E., Wind, C. A., and Waltman, S. R.: Validity of MacKay-Marg electronic applanation tonometer in patients with scarred irregular corneas. Am. J. Ophthalmol. 69:1003-1007, 1970. (The MacKay-Marg applanation tonometer is more reliable than the Goldmann device on diseased corneas.)

Kaufman, J. H., and Tolpin, D. W.: Glaucoma after traumatic angle recession. Am. J. Ophthalmol. 78:648-654, 1974. (A ten-year prospective study based on the population of the Howard, Hutchinson and Fredrick study resulted in only a 9% incidence of glaucoma.)

Kirsch, R. E., and Anderson, D. R.: Identification of the glaucomatous disc. Trans. Am. Acad. Ophthalmol. Otolaryngol. 77:143-156, 1973. (Increasing vertical ovality of the cup is an early sign of glaucoma.)

Kitazawa, Y., and Horie, T.: Diurnal variation of intraocular pressure in primary open-angle glaucoma. Am. J. Ophthalmol. 79:557-566, 1975. (Peak intraocular pressure occurs during the day rather than during early morning as previously described.)

Kronfeld, P. C.: The optic nerve. *In* Symposium on Glaucoma, 15th, 1966: Transactions of the New Orleans Academy of Ophthalmology. pp. 62-73. St. Louis, C. V. Mosby Co., 1967. (Observations of glaucomatous atrophy stemming from Elschnig normal disc types.)

————: The hypotensive action of anticholinesterases. A comparative study. Am. J. Ophthalmol. 61 (5/Part II): 258-264, 1966. (Phospholine iodide is the weakest and shortest acting of the long-acting cholinesterase inhibitors; humorosol is intermediate, and fluoropryl is the strongest and longest.)

Kupfer, C.: Clinical significance of pseudofacility. Am. J. Ophthalmol. 75:193-204, 1973. (One of the antiglaucomatous effects of pilocarpine and epinephrine, at least in young people, is a decrease in the formation of aqueous by means of ultrafiltration.)

Kupfer, C., Kuwabara, T., and Kaiser-Kupfer, M.: The histopathology of pigment dispersion syndrome with glaucoma. Am. J. Ophthalmol. 80:857-862, 1975. (This syndrome is apparently a congenital or developmental anomaly, and is characterized by a loss and thinning of outer iris epithelium as well as an increase in dilator muscle fibers; the coexistence of glaucoma is probably purely coincidental.)

Kurz, G. H.: Phacoanaphylactic endophthalmitis. Arch. Ophthalmol. 69:473-475, 1963. (Both the acute and the granulomatous cellular responses to a traumatically ruptured lens obstruct the aqueous outflow pathways.)

Lawrence, G. A.: Surgical treatment of patients with advanced glaucomatous field defects. Arch. Ophthalmol. 81:804-807, 1969. (Rapid loss of visual field did not occur after filtering surgery.)

Leydhecker, W.: The intraocular pressure: clinical aspects. Ann. Ophthalmol. 8:389-399, 1976. (Interobserver variation of Goldmann applanation tonometry is ±2.5 mm Hg; intraindividual error in reading Schiøtz tonometers is no greater than ±1 scale unit.)

Lichter, P. R.: Iris processes in 340 eyes. Am. J. Ophthalmol. 68:872-878, 1969. (Of normal eyes, 57% have iris processes, many of which insert anterior to the scleral spur.)

Lichter, P. R., and Shaffer, R. N.: Diagnostic and prognostic signs in pigmentary glaucoma. Trans. Am. Acad. Ophthalmol. Otolaryngol. 74:984-998, 1970. (Approximately one-quarter of patients don't have a Krukenberg spindle, a densely pigmented trabeculum, or myopia, and are neither young nor male.)

Palmberg, P. F., et al.: The reproducibility of the intraocular pressure response to dexamethasone. Am. J. Ophthalmol. 80:844-856, 1975. (Repeat steroid provocation in the same individuals has a response consistency of 75%.)

Perry, H. D., Yanoff, M., and Scheie, H. G.: Rubeosis in Fuchs heterochromic iridocyclitis. Arch. Ophthalmol. 93:337-339, 1975. (Both neovascularization of the angle and trabeculitis caused the glaucoma.)

Phelps, C. D., and Watzke, R. C.: Hemolytic glaucoma. Am. J. Ophthalmol. 80:690-695, 1975. (Irrigation of hemolytic debris can greatly improve this glaucoma.)

Podos, S. M., and Becker, B.: Tonography—current thoughts (editorial). Am. J. Ophthalmol. 75:733-735, 1973. (Tonography is an aid to glaucoma evaluation but not the basis for its diagnosis.)

Pohjanpelto, P. E.: The fellow eye in unilateral hypertensive pseudoexfoliation. Am. J. Ophthalmol. 75:216-220, 1973. (Ocular hypertension was found in 60% of the other eyes of patients with this supposedly unilateral disease.)

Pollack, I. P.: Diagnosis of the glaucomas. Pages 31-61. In Symposium on Glaucoma, 15th, 1966: Transactions of the New Orleans Academy of Ophthalmology, St. Louis, C. V. Mosby, Co., 1967. (A description of many clinical entities responsible for secondary glaucoma.)

Portney, G. L.: Photogrammetric analysis of the three dimensional geometry of normal and glaucomatous optic cups. Trans. Am. Acad. Ophthalmol. Otolaryngol. 81:239-246, 1976. (Quantitative descriptions of normal cup shapes and their presumed alterations from glaucoma.)

Quigley, H. A., Pollack, I. P., and Harbin, T. S., Jr.: Pilocarpine ocuserts. Arch. Ophthalmol. 93:771-775, 1975. (P-20 ocuserts have a level of effect similar to pilocarpine .5 to 1%; P-40 ocuserts are similar to pilocarpine 2 to 4%.)

Read, R. M., and Spaeth, G. L.: The practical clinical appraisal of the optic disc in glaucoma. Trans. Am. Acad Ophthalmol. Otolaryngol. 78:255-274, 1974. (Describes fives signs of glaucomatous disc change: polar notching, temporal unfolding, laminar dot sign, sharpened rim, and bayoneting at the disc edge; correlates these signs with the extent of visual field damage.)

Richardson, K. T.: Functional status of the glaucoma patient. Invest. Ophthalmol. 11:102-107, 1972. (Recommends placing patients in one of four categories and choosing the intensity of treatment based on the classification of each individual.)

Scheie, H. G.: Retraction of scleral wound edges. Am. J. Ophthalmol. 45 (4/part II):220-229, 1958. (A description of the thermosclerostomy.)

Schwartz, B.: Cupping and pallor of the optic disc. Arch. Ophthalmol. 89:272-277, 1973. (In glaucomatous eyes, there is usually more cupping than pallor.)

Schwartz, J. T., et al.: Twin study on ocular pressure following topically applied dexamethasone. II. Inheritance of variations in pressure response. Arch. Ophthalmol. 90:281-286, 1973 (Of monozygotic twins, 65% responded similarly to steroid provocation.)

Sears, M. L.: Surgical management of black ball hyphemas. Trans. Am. Acad. Ophthalmol. Otolaryngol. 74:820-827, 1970. (An anterior chamber clot can be expressed most easily on the fourth day after hemorrhage; earlier, it is insufficiently retracted; later, it is organized to adjacent tissues.)

van Herrick, W., Shaffer, R. N., and Schwartz, A:. Estimation of width of angle of anterior chamber. Am. J. Ophthalmol. 68:626-629, 1969. (Angle width is well correlated with the percentage of corneal slit thickness as seen with the slit lamp at the periphery of the anterior chamber; a wide open angle is recognized by being at least as wide as one corneal parallelipiped.)

Wadsworth, J. A. C.: Corneoscleral cautery—pathology and technique. Arch. Ophthalmol. 94:633-636, 1976. (Both the trephine and iridencleisis operations promote the sealing over of the scleral opening; the thermosclerotomy operation does not.)

Worthen, D. M.: Scanning electron microscopy after alpha chymotrypsin perfusion in man. Am. J. Ophthalmol. 73:637-642, 1972. (Broken and clumped zonules pass into the trabecular meshwork, where they block the outflow of aqueous.)

Zimmerman, T. J., and Worthen, D. M.: A comparison of two-hand applanation tonometers. Arch. Ophthalmol. 88:421-423, 1972. (The Perkins tonometer is easier to use than the Halberg because of the similarity of the former's design to that of the Goldmann tonometer.)

Chapter 3

ANGLE-CLOSURE GLAUCOMAS

DIAGNOSIS AND TREATMENT OF PRIMARY ANGLE-CLOSURE GLAUCOMA

Mechanism of Pupillary Block Glaucoma

The basic requirements of an acute attack of angle-closure glaucoma are: (1) a narrow anterior chamber angle; (2) pupillary block; (3) iris bombé.

In an eye with a sufficiently precarious narrow angle, the following events can occur (Fig. 3-1):

1. If the pupil dilates to a certain point where the iris is in increased contact with the lens (usually greatest at a diameter of 4 to 5 mm), the passage of aqueous from the posterior to the anterior chamber is retarded. This is called relative pupillary block. If almost no aqueous can pass through, the block is then nearly absolute.

2. Posterior pressure on the peripheral part of the iris builds up owing to the continued production of aqueous, which forces the peripheral iris to assume an anteriorly convex shape. This is called "iris bombé."

3. If the original chamber angle was already dangerously shallow, then the iris bombé can oppose the iris to the trabeculum, blocking most of the aqueous outflow. This complex mechanism causes the intraocular pressure to rise sharply.

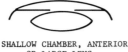

SHALLOW CHAMBER, ANTERIOR
OR LARGE LENS

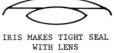

IRIS MAKES TIGHT SEAL
WITH LENS

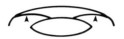

AQUEOUS TRANSIT THROUGH
PUPIL SLOWS, BUILDING UP
PRESSURE BEHIND IRIS

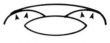

IRIDO-TRABECULAR CONTACT
OCCURS BLOCKING AQUEOUS
OUTFLOW

Fig. 3-1.   The development of pupillary block angle-closure glaucoma.

At the time of diagnosis of an acute attack of angle-closure glaucoma, the pupil will most likely be found in mid-dilation. This occurs because this is the position of greatest pupillary block and because the iris is "caught" there by the rising intraocular pressure, which paralyzes the sphincter and keeps the pupil from moving further. Small hyperopic eyes in which the tissues are relatively compacted and the lens is relatively anterior in position are particularly prone to the combination of conditions that lead to angle closure.

Another significant factor is the degree of tautness of the iris diaphragm. This varies with the individual but, generally speaking, the smaller the pupil the tauter the iris diaphragm. However, a lax iris may have broad contact with the lens even when the pupil is quite small, thus increasing the relative pupillary block. Iris bombé probably will not occur until the iris diaphragm tautness is decreased sufficiently to allow it to bow forward from the posterior pressure. This may be why acute attacks of angle-closure glaucoma are rarely seen with a small pupil. However, with the right degree of iris diaphragm laxity, an acute attack can occur in a patient with a very small pupil.

Acute Signs and Symptoms

The patient with this disease usually appears with blurred vision (probably with colored halos seen around lights), much pain in and around the eye, nausea, and perhaps vomiting. The eye is injected, the cornea is cloudy, the pupil is in mid-dilation, the anterior chamber is shallow, and the intraocular pressure is usually in the fifties or more. Frequently, with gonioscopy, some of the angle structures can be identified partly around their circumference but, many times, none can be seen at all.

Vision is reduced because of the corneal changes. Initially, this may be due to distortion of the lamellae, but eventually, under high enough intraocular pressure, aqueous is forced into the cornea which then becomes edematous. Colored halos occur because the cornea diffracts the light, breaking it up into the hues of the rainbow. If the attack is prolonged, bullous keratopathy can ensue because of the increased intraocular pressure, driving aqueous under the corneal epithelium.

Pain varies in degree from a mild fullness to severe pain. The pain follows the course of the fifth cranial nerve and may even initiate reflex pain above or below the periorbital area. An oculo-vagal reflex is believed to be responsible for the production of nausea, vomiting, bradycardia, and sweating that frequently accompany the acute attack.

Redness of the eye is due to passive venous congestion secondary to the increased intraocular pressure. Both iris and conjunctival blood vessels are swollen with blood.

While under the effects of high pressure, the already mid-dilated pupil becomes paralyzed and eventually damaged and cataractous change develops in the subcapsular lens epithelium. In advanced cases, the pupil may assume an oval shape and resist constriction by any drug.

Treatment of Acute Primary Angle-Closure Glaucoma

The objectives of treatment are reduction of the elevated intraocular pressure and prevention of its recurrence. The first treatment objective can be accomplished by the following:

1. Alternately applying one drop of pilocarpine 2% and one drop of eserine .25% (a short-acting cholinesterase inhibitor) topically every ten minutes for the first two hours. After the pressure has been controlled, a maintenance dose of pilocarpine 2% each hour is warranted.
2. Simultaneously injecting 500 mg of acetazolamide intravenously and beginning an oral dose of 250 mg q.i.d. with a loading dose of 500 mg.
3. Starting an intravenous drip of a systemic hyperosmotic (such as 20% mannitol, 1.5 gm per kg of body weight) if the pressure is not below 30 mm Hg after a few hours following administration of the other medications. The intraocular pressure will be normalized in most patients following these measures, and will remain normal until the second objective can be realized.

The second objective is met by performing a peripheral iridectomy, preferably basally, which allows the aqueous access to the anterior chamber by a pathway other than through the pupil. This can be done with least complication by operating on a relatively quiet, normotensive eye that is no longer severely inflamed. For this reason, if possible, one should wait at least 48 hours after pressure normalization before undertaking this surgery.

In patients with aphakic pupillary block and resultant acute angle-closure glaucoma, argon laser iridotomy may be possible and serves the same purpose as iridectomy. Longer and stronger bursts of energy are needed in thick, brown irides in comparison with blue or atrophic irides. Many times, laser iridotomy in dark eyes is impossible.

Occasionally, the intraocular pressure will not remain

lowered long enough to allow this rest period without administering hyperosmotic agents, so that it may be necessary to reinstate mannitol therapy. The operation should then be performed after renormalization of pressure.

In cases of acute angle-closure glaucoma, one should institute treatment of the fellow eye with pilocarpine 1% q.i.d. immediately to prevent a similar episode there.

The hyperosmotic dehydrating agent oral glycerol should not be disregarded in the management of the acute attack. However, it cannot always be used successfully in a nauseated, vomiting patient because of its own potentially nauseating sweetness. Otherwise, it has great value, and should be used in 50% solution mixed with a sour juice in doses of 1 ml per pound of body weight.

Chronic Primary Angle-Closure Glaucoma

This form of glaucoma is caused by chronic obstruction of the angle in variable amounts; the symptoms run the gamut from virtually none (like primary open-angle) to intermittent spikes of sharp pain accompanied by mild congestion and colored halo formation. Actually, the contact between iris and trabeculum increases gradually, usually starting superiorly. No synechiae may be present when there is no congestion because, without it, there is no fibrous exudate to form synechiae. When the angle has closed sufficiently, the pressure begins to rise gradually and may reach levels of 40 to 60 mm Hg. Some synechiae may form late in the disease, but these may become obvious only after peripheral iridectomy relieves the posterior pressure on the iris. Iridectomy is the treatment of choice.

Gonioscopy is particularly important in this disease. A person with a pressure reading in the thirties may actually have chronic primary open-angle glaucoma, which may be overlooked unless careful gonioscopy is performed. In this case, a surgical "cure" by iridectomy is entirely possible if advanced synechia formation has not occurred.

Use of the Filtering Procedure

After an increase of intraocular pressure into the fifties or greater for more than 24 hours, some anterior synechiae may have begun to form. In a chronic primary angle-closure glaucoma patient with chronic pressure elevation or intermittent spikes of high pressure, the same events may have occurred. On this assumption, some ophthalmologists would be tempted to filter the eye in a single procedure combined with iridectomy. For those who would be so inclined, tonography can be somewhat useful for detecting an eye with reduced outflow after the pressure has been medically controlled. However, tonography is not always useful clinically and assumptions based on it are frequently less so. Gonioscopy at the time of surgery can be helpful because, after iridectomy, the chamber will automatically deepen or become deeper with irrigation, whereupon anterior synechiae can be seen easily. If a large area of the trabecular meshwork is occluded by these synechiae, then an immediate filtering procedure would be in order. If peripheral iridectomy alone is done and the pressure remains elevated postoperatively, the patient can be treated as one having primary open-angle glaucoma, first using medical therapy and then resorting to filtering surgery only when absolutely necessary. Even in the face of visual field loss, which infrequently occurs from an acute attack of primary angle-closure glaucoma, many patients recover remarkably well.

Evaluation of the Optic Disc and Visual Field

After an attack of acute angle-closure glaucoma, the likelihood of a patient having a normal optic disc or field is greater than 60%. In contrast, those with chronic primary angle-closure glaucoma more closely parallel patients with primary open-angle glaucoma with regard to their glaucomatous damage. The duration of the pressure elevation, therefore, seems to be directly correlated with the presence of disc and visual field changes, but the height of the pressure rise is not.

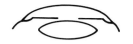

CHAMBER DEEP CENTRALLY WHERE
IRIS "PLATEAUS" BUT ANGLE IS
NARROW

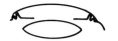

WHEN IRIS DILATES IT BUNCHES UP
IN A NARROW ANGLE AND CONTACTS
WITH TRABECULAR MESHWORK

Fig. 3-2. The development of nonpupillary block angle-closure glaucoma.

Angle-Closure Glaucoma Without Pupillary Block

This is an anatomic problem in which the anterior chamber is not necessarily shallower than normal and pupillary block is only a small component of the disease. The mechanism of an acute attack of this form of primary angle-closure glaucoma is the bunching of peripheral iris against the trabeculum (Fig. 3-2.) The gonioscopic picture is one of a plateau iris, wherein the angle between peripheral iris and cornea is acute but the iris "plateaus off" sharply just after the trabecular zone. An acute attack can occur without dilation by medications, although such mydriasis is a common initial cause. Because of the minimal pupillary block coupled with the need to remove as much basal iris as is practical, a broad basal peripheral iridectomy or even multiple iridectomies should be performed. Unfortunately, dilation of the pupil afterwards could still provoke an acute attack in such a patient. In some cases, however, the surgical procedure completely solves the problem.

DIAGNOSIS AND TREATMENT OF SECONDARY ANGLE-CLOSURE GLAUCOMA

As in open-angle disease, the limitations imposed by the primary processes are most important.

With Pupillary Block

In lens-induced glaucoma, a swollen hypermature lens or anterior lens dislocation can obstruct the flow of aqueous.

These problems are easily relieved by treating the patient with the standard medical approach to an acute attack of primary angle-closure glaucoma, followed shortly thereafter by lens extraction. In the case of anterior lens dislocation into the anterior chamber, great care should be taken to prevent losing the lens into the vitreous. This can be accomplished most easily by medically constricting the pupil and trapping the lens in front of the iris.

Posterior synechiae can occur in either phakic or aphakic eyes of uveitic patients. If the synechiae are sufficient in number to cause a secluded pupil, true iris bombé will result. If vigorous attempts at dilating the pupil fail to break the posterior synechiae, peripheral iridectomy is indicated after medical reduction of the intraocular pressure.

Without Pupillary block

Anterior synechiae can develop after a long-standing iritis, or if a flat anterior chamber persists for more than a few days. Medical and surgical treatment as for primary open-angle glaucoma is indicated, because the iris is so adherent to the trabeculum that peripheral iridectomy will do little or nothing to improve the outflow.

Neovascular membrane formation frequently occurs in conjunction with rubeosis iridis. As the membrane shrinks, the angle closes. Treatment as in primary open-angle glaucoma is necessary for the same reason as exists with anterior synechiae.

MALIGNANT GLAUCOMA

This is a rare but dreaded form of secondary angle-closure glaucoma. It can occur after a filtering procedure for glaucoma or even after iridectomy alone, especially for chronic primary angle-closure glaucoma. Initially, the lens moves forward, possibly due to lax zonules, which brings it into contact with the ciliary body and blocks the normal aqueous movement from the posterior to the anterior chamber. Pressure then builds up posterior to the ciliary body, owing to the ciliary block, followed by iris bombé and then angle-closure with increased intraocular pressure.

Therapy is directed toward relaxing the ciliary body and flattening it out with topical atropine, thereby opening a space between the lens and the ciliary body. Hyperosmotic agents may break the acute attack by allowing the lens to fall back, but lens extraction is usually necessary because, after discontinuing this therapy, another attack would probably ensue when the vitreous rehydrates. In some cases, vitreous drainage plus repeat iridectomy have been curative without lens extraction. In others, the chronic administration of atropine has appeared to solve the problem.

COMBINED MECHANISM GLAUCOMA

Although the categories of primary and secondary glaucoma are well defined, some patients may have a combination of glaucoma types. The combinations are four possible arrangements, the secondary process being any one of the many already discussed:

1. primary open-primary closure
2. primary open-secondary closure
3. secondary open-primary closure
4. secondary open-secondary closure

A patient with an angle-closure component caused by pupillary block can be helped by peripheral iridectomy. On the other hand, the open-angle component must be treated in its standard fashion. The challenge in these cases is to unravel the components of the disease, determine exactly the extent to which the narrowness of a particular angle influences the glaucoma, and decide on the appropriate therapy. In particular, the combination of chronic primary angle-closure glaucoma and primary open-angle glaucoma is certainly one of the most challenging diagnoses in all of ophthalmology.

GONIOSCOPICALLY NARROW ANGLES

In an eye in which no symptoms or signs of angle-closure glaucoma have occurred but there is a worrisome narrow angle, the following tests can be used. However, they are not essential because careful gonioscopy alone should be sufficient to make a therapeutic decision.

Dark-Room Provocative Test. The patient remains awake in a dark room for 60 to 90 minutes. A positive test consists of finding an increase of 8 mm Hg in intraocular pressure in association with semi-dilated pupils *and* a closed angle upon gonioscopy.

Prone Provocative Test. The patient lies in a prone position for 60 minutes, after which tonometry and gonioscopy are performed. In a positive test, the intraocular pressure is elevated 8 mm Hg or more and gonioscopy reveals a closed angle.

In both these tests, it is difficult to identify a closed angle because the light source for gonioscopy causes rapid miosis or the change to an upright or supine position for gonioscopy causes the iris to fall away from the trabeculum.

Mydriatic Provocative Test. Instillation of 1% paredrine in *one eye only* should produce moderate dilation within 45 minutes. A positive test is a rise in intraocular pressure of 8 mm Hg and a closed angle upon gonioscopy.

If any of these tests are positive, miotics should then be instilled immediately and pilocarpine 1% q.i.d. prescribed. However, peripheral iridectomy should not be performed on the basis of these tests alone. When one eye is positive, the other eye should also be treated with pilocarpine even if its tests were negative. A negative test in both eyes does not mean that an angle-closure attack cannot occur, but only suggests that the patient might be watched closely without therapy.

Other Considerations. Of course, a variety of factors can alter this approach. Performing gonioscopy on a patient who is receiving prophylactic pilocarpine to ascertain the degree of openness of the angle can be most helpful in determining the effectiveness of medication. Increasing nuclear sclerosis may reduce vision following miotics so that iridectomy may become necessary sooner than otherwise anticipated. Perhaps the lens may require extraction, thereby solving visual and pressure problems.

In any event, close observation of all patients suspected of developing primary angle-closure glaucoma is important. Remember that, for some unknown reason, pupillary block is more likely to occur when the pupil is in mid-dilation rather than at its maximum. Furthermore, this happens more frequently when the pupil is coming down after mydriasis than when it is enlarging. Areas of closed angle are found most often superiorly and least often inferiorly. Approximately 50% of the angle or more must be closed before the pressure will rise to the levels ordinarily seen in acute primary angle-closure glaucoma. All of these factors must be considered in determining the proper approach to each patient's care, because a negative provocative test is not a guarantee that an acute attack of primary angle-closure glaucoma cannot occur.

SUGGESTED READINGS

Anderson, D. R., Forster, R. K., and Lewis, M. L.: Laser iridotomy for aphakic pupillary block. Arch. Ophthalmol. 93:343-346, 1975. (Hazardous in phakic patients due to the possibility of damage to the lens, which might occur from the necessarily strong and long energy levels that are required for complete penetration of the iris.)

Becker, B., and Thompson, H. E.: Tonography and angle-closure glaucoma: Diagnosis and therapy. Am. J. Ophthalmol. 46:305-310, 1958. (Tonography can be used to differentiate eyes with low outflow which are in need of filtration from those with normal outflow which can be cured by iridectomy alone.)

Bhargava, S. K., Leighton, D. A., and Phillips, C. I.: Early angle-closure glaucoma. Arch. Ophthalmol. 89:369-372, 1973. (Closed angles are most commonly found superiorly, whether due to synechiae or iridotrabecular apposition.)

Chandler, P.A.: Choice of treatment in dislocation of the lens. Arch. Ophthalmol. 71:765-786, 1964. (Anterior lens dislocation may not cause the lens to prolapse into the anterior chamber but, instead, may allow it to move into posterior contact with the pupil, which it blocks; this leads to the formation of peripheral anterior synechiae and chronic angle-closure if not treated early.)

————: Narrow-angle glaucoma. Arch. Ophthalmol. 47:695-716, 1952. (A complete description of the pathogenesis, signs, and treatment of angle-closure glaucoma.)

Chandler, P. A., and Grant, W. M.: Mydriatic-cycloplegic treatment in malignant glaucoma. Arch. Ophthalmol. 68:353-359, 1962. (Malignant glaucoma occurs only in eyes in which surgical procedures are performed when the angle is closed or the pressure is elevated; it is not relieved by glaucoma surgery. Miotics worsen the condition, but cycloplegics make the zonules taut and pull the lens into a normal position.)

Chandler, P. A., and Trotter, R. R.: Angle-closure glaucoma: Subacute types. Arch. Ophthalmol. 53:305-317, 1955. (Pressure increase is less than in acute closure, and most eyes are "normal" between attacks; early iridectomy is advised before many synechiae form.)

Douglas, G. R., Drance, S. M., and Schulzer, M.: The visual field and nerve head in angle-closure glaucoma. Arch. Ophthalmol. 93:409-411, 1975. (Cupping is more common in chronic angle-closure glaucoma than in the acute disease, perhaps owing to the increased duration of pressure elevation in the former.)

Drance, S. M.: Effect of oral glycerol on intraocular pressure in normal and glaucomatous eyes. Arch. Ophthalmol. 72:491-493, 1964. (Causes intraocular pressure to drop almost as much as intravenous hyperosmotic agents.)

Foulds, W. S.: Observations on the darkroom test and its mechanism. Brit. J. Ophthalmol. 41:200-207, 1957. (Of known angle-closure eyes, 56% reponded positively to dark provocation; the higher the pretest pressure, the greater the magnitude of its elevation.)

Harris, L. S., and Galin, M. A.: Prone provocative testing for narrow angle glaucoma. Arch. Ophthalmol. 87:493-496, 1972. (Placing an eye in a prone position causes the iris to come in closer contact with the trabeculum and the lens with the pupil; when this test is combined with dark provocation, 90% of patients with narrow angles have a positive response.)

Kirsch, R. E.: A study of provocative tests for angle closure glaucoma. Arch. Ophthalmol. 74:770-776, 1965. (The essence of a positive provocative test for angle closure is its ability to increase pupillary block; this is best done when mydriasis, water drinking, and miosis are done sequentially and together.)

Kronfeld, P. C.: Angle-closure glaucoma. Trans. Am. Acad. Ophthalmol. Otolaryngol. 67:476-482, 1963. (Operating room gonioscopy and preoperative tonography are important adjuncts to determining which type of surgery to perform.)

Lowe, R. F.: Angle-closure, pupil dilatation, and pupil block. Brit. J. Ophthalmol. 50:385-389, 1966. (Pupillary block is more likely to occur with mydriatics than with cycloplegics, although the effects of cycloplegics are more easily reversible.)

Mapstone, R.: Mechanics of pupil block. Brit. J. Ophthalmol. 52:19-25, 1968. (Pupillary block is due to the force of the dilator and the stretching of the iris, which are enhanced by an anteriorly placed lens; alpha-adrenergic drugs are more capable of beneficially correcting the balance of forces in such an eye than are parasympathomimetics.)

Pollack, I. P.: Chronic angle-closure glaucoma. Arch. Ophthalmol. 85:676-689, 1971. (Initially there may be no symptoms of angle closure and no pressure rise with mydriasis; the diagnosis rests on the gonioscopic findings.)

Shaffer, R. N.: A suggested anatomic classification to define the pupillary block glaucomas. Invest. Ophthalmol. 12:540-542, 1973. (Iridolenticular block is suggested for posterior synechiae to the lens; iridovitreal block for posterior synechiae to the vitreous.)

————: Open-angle glaucoma. Trans. Am. Acad. Ophthalmol. Otolaryngol. 67:467-475, 1963. (In some young patients with open angles, the symptoms of acute primary angle-closure glaucoma can occur due to sharp peaks in pressure; on the other hand, subacute angle closure can appear symptomatically like open-angle glaucoma.)

————: Gonioscopy, ophthalmoscopy and perimetry. Trans. Am. Acad. Ophthalmol. Otolaryngol. 64:112-127, 1960. (Eyes with plateau irides do not have particularly shallow anterior chambers, so that gonioscopy might be inadvertently neglected in a symptomless patient.)

————: Operating room gonioscopy in angle-closure glaucoma surgery. Arch. Ophthalmol. 59:532-535, 1958. (Fill the anterior chamber with saline and use the Koeppe lens to determine the extent of the anterior synechiae.)

Tomlinson, A., and Leighton, D. A.: Ocular dimensions in the heredity of angle-closure glaucoma. Brit. J. Ophthalmol. 57:475-486, 1973. (A-scan ultrasonic measurements on the eyes of patients with iridectomies after angle-closure glaucoma were compared with normal eyes; in the former, the anterior chamber was shallower, the lens was thicker, and the axial length was smaller.)

Weiss, D. I., and Shaffer, R. N.: Ciliary block (malignant) glaucoma. Trans. Am. Acad. Ophthalmol. Otolaryngol. 76:450-461, 1972. (The etiology of malignant glaucoma is ciliolenticular block in phakic eyes and ciliovitreal block in aphakic eyes.)

Weiss, D. I., Shaffer, R. N., and Wise, B. L.: Mannitol infusion to reduce intraocular pressure. Arch. Ophthalmol. 68:341-347, 1962. (An effective treatment that should be used cautiously in patients with cardiac, vascular, or renal disease.)

Chapter 4

CONGENITAL GLAUCOMAS

Definition

Congenital glaucoma is a broad term that is used to describe glaucomas that occur prior to middle age and may be associated with ocular anomalies, extraocular abnormalities, and syndromes. Those that are not can be categorized as primary infantile glaucoma. Nearly all of these diseases are genetically determined and are caused by an obstruction to outflow.

Gonioscopic Appearance

In some of these angles, a specific structure that is believed to restrict access of aqueous to the trabeculum can be seen. For example, in neurofibromatosis, an irregular, avascular, lightly pigmented tissue may be present in the angle along with a scattering of nodules. However, most of these diseases gonioscopically resemble primary infantile glaucoma. In this disease, the iris inserts directly into the trabecular surface, which is unusually condensed into a quasimembrane (Barkan's). As a result, there is no apparent angle recess, but rather, the iris stroma rises gradually and the peripheral vasculature slopes upward to meet the uveal meshwork. The ciliary body is barely visible through the thick, gelatinous-like substance of the unusually broad trabecular band.

The incision of Barkan's membrane by goniotomy is believed to allow successful egress of aqueous and normalization of intraocular pressure.

Signs and Symptoms of Primary Infantile Glaucoma

If the disease becomes manifest in the first year after birth, then lacrimation, photophobia, and blepharospasm may be present. However, the finding of increased intraocular pressure coupled with corneal edema, corneal enlargement, and tears in Descemet's membrane are most specific diagnostically. After age 3, these signs are infrequent, which might allow the glaucoma to progress unnoticed. Further confusion can result from the use of most general anesthetics, which falsely lower the intraocular pressure. Ketamine, on the other hand, raises it. Therefore, if the ocular tension is abnormally elevated under the influence of inhalation anesthesia, glaucoma is a likely diagnosis. If the pressure is normal under ketamine, glaucoma is probably not present.

Of great importance is the observation of cupping of the optic nerve head, which is particularly prominent in the 25% of cases in whom this disease is monocular; cupping seems to occur earlier in children with glaucoma than in adults. For both funduscopy and simultaneous gonioscopy of the infant, the smooth-domed Koeppe lens is particulary valuable.

Treatment

In early infantile glaucoma, goniotomy is the treatment of choice if the angle can be visualized. If not, trabeculotomy ab externo should be employed. Goniopuncture is another procedure to consider, but it does not appear to have a potential for long-term control of intraocular pressure.

In late-developing infantile glaucoma, medical management should be attempted before resorting to surgery. If this fails, trabeculectomy should be attempted rather than goniotomy, which is less reliable in older children. This form of external fistulization can also be used for patients who have not responded to multiple goniotomies for the control of early infantile glaucoma.

SUGGESTED READINGS

Scheie, H. G.: Goniopuncture—A new filtering operation for glaucoma. Arch. Ophthalmol. 44:761-782, 1950. (A description of the technique.)

Shaffer, R. N.: Goniotomy technique in congenital glaucoma. Am. J. Ophthalmol. 47:90-97, 1959, (A description of the technique.)

Shaffer, R. N., and Hetherington, J.: The glaucomatous disc in infants. Trans. Am. Acad. Ophthalmol. Otolaryngol. 73:929-935, 1969. (Cupping can occur without interference with optic nerve function and can disappear after pressure normalization.)

Waring, G. O., Rodrigues, M. M., and Laibson, P. R.: Anterior chamber cleavage syndrome. A stepladder classification. Surv. Ophthalmol. 20:3-27, 1975. (Describes the gonioscopic and histopathologic findings in Axenfeld's anomaly, Rieger's anomaly, iridogoniodysgenesis, Peter's anomaly, and anterior chamber cleavage syndrome, all of which may have congenital or developmental glaucoma.)

Weiss, D. I., Cooper, L. Z., and Green, R. H.: Infantile glaucoma—a manifestation of congenital rubella. JAMA 195:725-727, 1966. (In one case, glaucoma was delayed until the eighth month; in two cases, it occurred in one eye only.)

Section II

CLINICAL EXAMINATION METHODS

Chapter 5

TECHNIQUE OF PROJECTION PERIMETRY

The complete examination of a visual field is a time-consuming task. In fact, one method of static perimetry that makes use of two different perimeters requires one and one-half hours per eye. Theoretically, this technique will uncover the vast majority of visual field defects, but some may still be missed. Kinetic perimetry, in contrast to this static technique, requires less time but is even less capable of identifying all existing scotomas. Nevertheless, it is the most common mode of visual field testing and has been significantly improved by the advent of projection perimeters. The Haag-Streit Goldmann machine is the prototype of such instruments (Figs. 5-1, 5-2, 5-3); its specifications are described in the section on diagnosis and therapy.

GOLDMANN PERIMETER

To use the Goldmann perimeter properly, one must calibrate it daily. This is done by directing the 64 mm²/1000 asb target (V/4) onto the light meter located on the side of the instrument, and then adjusting the rheostat so that the meter reads 1000 asb. The white flag is then lowered into the same location as the light meter and a 64 mm²/31.5 asb target (V/1) is used to illuminate it. The housing on the projection bulb is then manually adjusted so that the intensity of light on the flag matches its surroundings. A background illumination of 31.5 asb is thereby achieved.

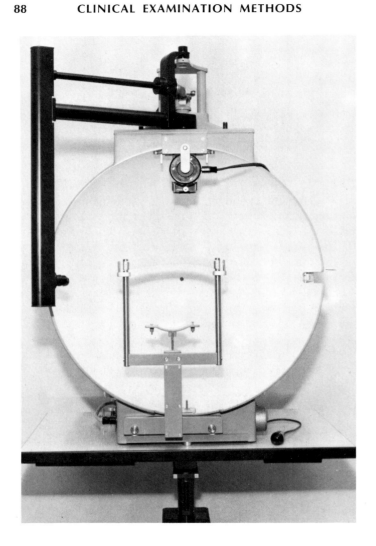

Fig. 5-1. Patient's view of the Goldmann Perimeter.

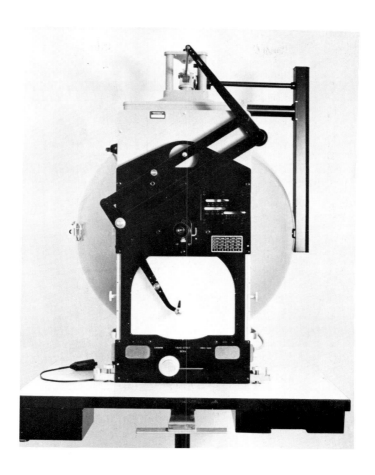

Fig. 5-2.   Examiner's view of the Goldmann Perimeter.

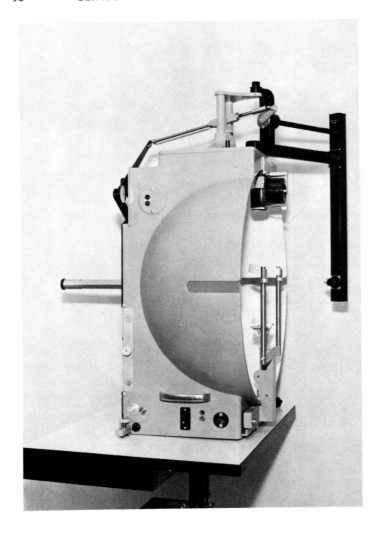

Fig. 5-3. Side view of the Goldmann Perimeter.

Chart 5-1. Before Starting Perimetry

1. Calibrate the target and background luminance of the dome.
2. Make certain that the pupil is 3 mm or larger.
3. Determine the proper refraction for 30-cm distance.
4. Line up the patient's pupil in the fixation telescope.
5. Allow five minutes for the patient to adapt to the background luminance of the perimeter.

Before beginning the examination, check the patient's pupils. Unless they are fully reactive to light or at least 3 mm or larger, it is best to dilate the pupil, as long as there is no contraindication. Miotic pupils can artificially constrict the visual field and induce scotomas. In contrast, large fixed pupils do not seem to influence the results of perimetry negatively. Moreover, visual field tests should be performed with the pupil at nearly the same diameter each time, so that results can be reliably compared in subsequent examinations.

The refraction for a distance of 30 cm should also be checked before proceeding. It is essential to have the best corrected acuity each time the central visual field is tested, for the same reason that it is important to control the pupil size. If the distance correction is known, then Goldmann's table for the amount of sphere to be added at 30 cm may be used (Table

Table 5-1. Goldmann's Recommended* Spectacle Addition for 30 cm. Testing Distance

Age	Sphere
30-40 yrs	+1.00
40-45 yrs	+1.50
45-50 yrs	+2.00
50-55 yrs	+2.50
Over 55 yrs	+3.25

*Haag-Streit Goldmann Perimeter 940. Instructions: Assembly, Use and Maintenance. Berne, Switzerland.

5-1). If the pupil has been dilated with cycloplegic agents, +3.25 will be needed in addition to the refraction required for distance, even if the pupil enlarges only a few millimeters. To minimize the number of lenses in the holder, the refractive spherical equivalent may be used, unless there is marked astigmatism. Lenses with small rims are desirable to avoid producing a false scotoma, which any lens can produce at its edge. In fact, when examining the field near the 30 degree radius, special care must be taken to avoid this problem by removing the lens whenever its rim blocks the view of the target.

The room should be tight from light from other sources and the patient should be given five minutes to adapt to the background luminance of the dome. Meanwhile, he should be familiarized with the response pushbutton and become comfortably seated with his chin and forehead against their rests. His head position should be adjusted so that fixation is central and can be continually monitored by the perimetrist during the examination by sighting the pupil through the telescope orifice in the dome.

ROUTINE VISUAL FIELD TESTING (KINETIC AND SUPRATHRESHOLD STATIC PERIMETRY)

Presentation Patterns

Begin the examination without the corrective lens and gradually bring a 1 mm²/1000 asb target (II/4e) in from the periphery at a rate of 5 degrees/second on the 45-, 135-, 225-, and 315-degree meridians in order to familiarize the patient with the procedure (Fig. 5-4). Ask him to respond when he first sees the target and make certain that he understands that he should signal only when the target first appears. Also remind him to keep his head position stable and maintain fixation at all times.

If the patient cannot see the target on any of the four pretest meridians, check to be sure that his nose is not blocking his

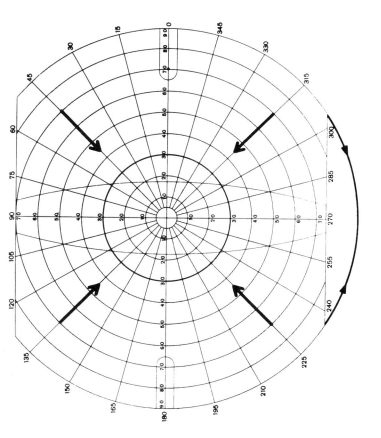

Fig. 5-4. Familiarization phase of radial kinetic perimetry on the 45-, 135-, 225-, and 315-degree meridians.

93

Chart 5-2. Routine Visual Field Testing

1. Basic kinetic examination maps isopter borders in two directions:
    a. radial movement inward along the major meridians to measure their length.
    b. circular movement along circumferential arc(s) to identify the extent of wedges or nasal steps at the isopter boundary.
2. Static spot checks determine the approximate sensitivity of regions between isopters.
3. Kinetic scotoma mapping plots the area of all scotomas, including the blind spot, using a radial movement outward from their centers.

---

nasal field and that his lid is not drooping and blocking his superior field. In either case, his head can be rotated slightly to keep the nose out of the way or his lid can be taped up. If neither adjustment alters the patient's response, use the 64 mm²/1000 asb target (V/4e) and begin again.

From this juncture, the presentation of the target should follow one of four patterns, chosen as needed:

1. basic kinetic examination
    a. radial presentation
    b. circular presentation
2. static spot checks
3. kinetic scotoma mapping

Basic Kinetic Examination. At least four different isopters should be plotted. The selection of the appropriate target size and the luminance to use for these isopters are described on page 101.

Radial Presentation. Move the target in from the periphery toward fixation along each of 24 meridians, which are spaced at 15 degree intervals (Fig. 5-5), and proceed in a counter-clockwise manner starting at 15 degrees for the right eye and 195 degrees for the left. Record the location where the target is first seen. This is the radius of that meridian.

If one meridian (or more) is 10 degrees or more shorter than the others, recheck the short meridian(s), using the same

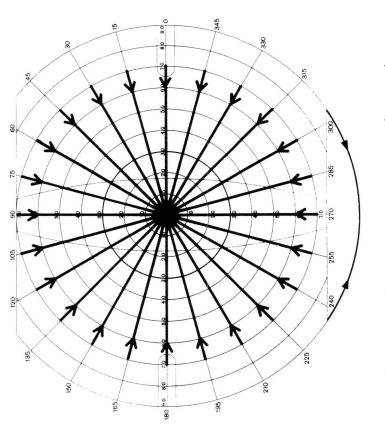

Fig. 5-5. Radial kinetic perimetry on 24 major meridians spaced at 15-degree intervals.

technique as above. If it is verified to be at least 10 degrees shorter than the other meridians, circular kinetic perimetry should be done to determine the exact pattern of the irregularly shaped isopter.

Once the isopter radius comes to 30 degrees in any quadrant, it is necessary to place the proper spectacle correction in the lens holder before mapping anything inside this radius.

Circular Presentation. Test the field with the same stimulus that was originally used to find the length of the meridians, moving the target in a circular manner from the short meridian that is farthest away from the long meridian (Fig. 5-6). Use an arc that is slightly greater in radius than that of the short meridian (for consistency, choose a radius half-way between those of the short and long meridians). The field should be checked in both directions. In dealing with a possible nasal step, double- and triple-check this area by moving the target circularly toward the step at radial intervals of no more than 5 degrees (Fig. 5-7).

Static Spot Checks. Each time an isopter is mapped after the first one, static spot checks should be made between the newly plotted isopter and the last previously plotted isopter, using the target that was used to map the larger isopter. Also spot-check down to the 5 degree radius inside the most central isopter, using its target as the stimulus. Check at the intersection of each 15 degree meridian and each 5 degree radial interval (Fig. 5-8) by exposing the target for up to one second and asking the patient to respond when he sees it. The shutter dial on the side of the perimeter can be depressed for that period of time in order to turn on the target. When it is released, the target will automatically disappear. Recheck each missed point once before recording it.

Kinetic Scotoma Search. After a single or a group of spots is missed, the boundaries of the scotoma should be delineated by moving the missed target in a radial manner outward along eight meridians spaced 45 degrees apart, starting at the center

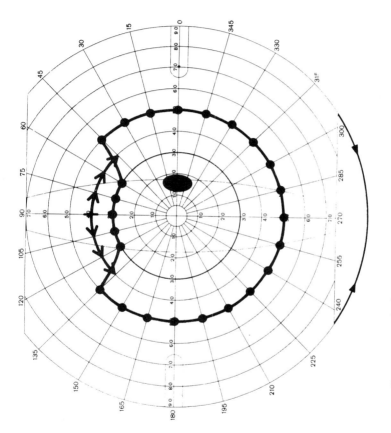

Fig. 5-6. Circular kinetic perimetry near a constricted portion of an isopter.

97

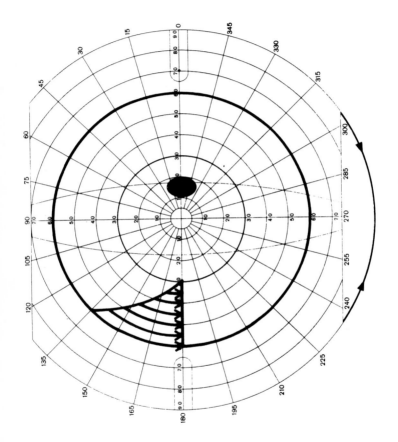

Fig. 5-7. Circular kinetic search for a nasal step.

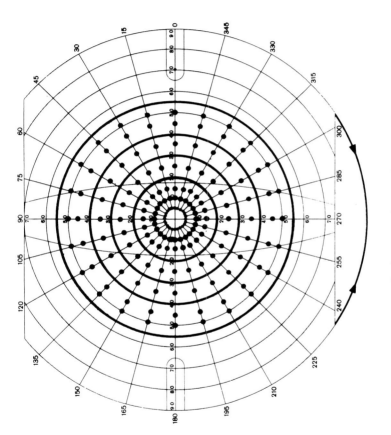

Fig. 5-8. Static spot check positions between isopters.

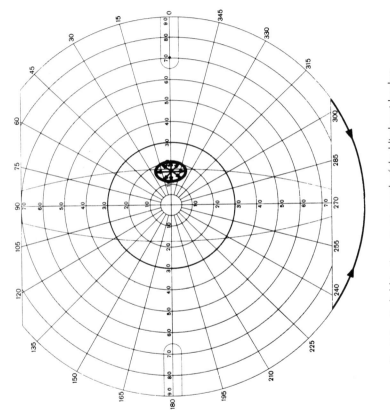

Fig. 5-9. Radial kinetic scotoma search of the blind spot borders.

of the missed point(s) (Fig. 5-9). After plotting the boundaries, increase the stimulus by one step, as described in the following protocol, and repeat the testing.

The blind spot should be plotted in the same manner, using the target stimulus that mapped the isopter whose radius is 30 degrees on the temporal side. The blind spot should also be plotted with the target that was used to map an isopter that had approximately 20 degrees of temporal radius.

It is helpful to use a color-coded system for connecting the marks that are made in response to the same stimulus values. For example, if red is used for the 1/4 mm²/1000 asb target (I/2e), then the isopter produced with it should be red and the blind spot and any scotomas should be solidly colored in red as well. Any set of colors may be used, as long as they are consistent from time to time and from patient to patient.

Target Choices and Filter Characteristics

The approach to choosing the proper stimulus values is based on the goal of finishing the examination with isopters whose spacing does not exceed 15 degrees in the periphery or 10 degrees in the center (inside 30-degree radius). Furthermore, the beginning target should be selected so that the entire peripheral field can be mapped with it. For most people, this is the 1 mm²/1000 asb target (II/4e). If, during the familiarization procedure, the patient cannot see this target at a radius of at least 45 degrees in all four preliminary meridians, the stimulus should be increased by one full step at a time (Table 5-2) until he can identify the target at 45 degrees

Chart 5-3. Deciding Which Targets to Use

1. Try to pick targets so that the spacing between isopters is no closer than 15 degrees in the periphery and 10 degrees centrally.
2. Use full- and half-step stimulus changes as guides (Tables 5-2 and 5-3).
3. Attempt to master the target filter system to make choices more conveniently.

Table 5-2.   Full-step Changes in Target Stimulus Value

Notation	Target
$\dfrac{\text{V}}{\text{4e}}$	$\dfrac{64 \text{ mm}^2}{1000 \text{ asb}}$
$\dfrac{\text{IV}}{\text{4e}}$	$\dfrac{16 \text{ mm}^2}{1000 \text{ asb}}$
$\dfrac{\text{III}}{\text{4e}}$	$\dfrac{4 \text{ mm}^2}{1000 \text{ asb}}$
$\dfrac{\text{II}}{\text{4e}}$	$\dfrac{1 \text{ mm}^2}{1000 \text{ asb}}$
$\dfrac{\text{I}}{\text{4e}}$	$\dfrac{\frac{1}{4} \text{ mm}^2}{1000 \text{ asb}}$
$\dfrac{\text{I}}{\text{3e}}$	$\dfrac{\frac{1}{4} \text{ mm}^2}{315 \text{ asb}}$
$\dfrac{\text{I}}{\text{2e}}$	$\dfrac{\frac{1}{4} \text{ mm}^2}{100 \text{ asb}}$
$\dfrac{\text{I}}{\text{1e}}$	$\dfrac{\frac{1}{4} \text{ mm}^2}{31.5 \text{ asb}}$

or beyond on all four meridians, or until the 64 mm²/1000 asb (V/4e) level is reached.

Once the appropriate peripheral target is found, decrease the stimulus by one full step at a time to map all the required isopters, spaced as described above. This may occasionally require the use of a target that is half-way in stimulus value between two full steps. To accomplish this, a .63 filter (c) can be put in place of the 1.00 filter (e), while continuing to use the particular size filter (Roman numerals 0 through V) and major luminance filter (Arabic numerals 1 through 4) that were employed to map the immediately larger isopter (Table 5-3.)

Rather than mapping an entire isopter before checking whether it is at a sufficient distance from the previous one, it is

Table 5-3.   Half-step Changes in Target Stimulus Value

Notation		Target	
$\dfrac{V}{4e}$		$\dfrac{64 \text{ mm}^2}{1000 \text{ asb}}$	
	$\dfrac{V}{4c}$		$\dfrac{64 \text{ mm}^2}{630 \text{ asb}}$
$\dfrac{IV}{4e}$		$\dfrac{16 \text{ mm}^2}{1000 \text{ asb}}$	
	$\dfrac{IV}{4c}$		$\dfrac{16 \text{ mm}^2}{630 \text{ asb}}$
$\dfrac{III}{4e}$		$\dfrac{4 \text{ mm}^2}{1000 \text{ asb}}$	
	$\dfrac{III}{4c}$		$\dfrac{4 \text{ mm}^2}{630 \text{ asb}}$
$\dfrac{II}{4e}$		$\dfrac{1 \text{ mm}^2}{1000 \text{ asb}}$	
	$\dfrac{II}{4c}$		$\dfrac{1 \text{ mm}^2}{630 \text{ asb}}$
$\dfrac{I}{4e}$		$\dfrac{\frac{1}{4} \text{ mm}^2}{1000 \text{ asb}}$	
	$\dfrac{I}{4c}$		$\dfrac{\frac{1}{4} \text{ mm}^2}{630 \text{ asb}}$
$\dfrac{I}{3e}$		$\dfrac{\frac{1}{4} \text{ mm}^2}{315 \text{ asb}}$	
	$\dfrac{I}{3c}$		$\dfrac{\frac{1}{4} \text{ mm}^2}{200 \text{ asb}}$
$\dfrac{I}{2e}$		$\dfrac{\frac{1}{4} \text{ mm}^2}{100 \text{ asb}}$	
	$\dfrac{I}{2c}$		$\dfrac{\frac{1}{4} \text{ mm}^2}{63 \text{ asb}}$
$\dfrac{I}{1e}$		$\dfrac{\frac{1}{4} \text{ mm}^2}{31.5 \text{ asb}}$	
	$\dfrac{I}{1c}$		$\dfrac{\frac{1}{4} \text{ mm}^2}{20 \text{ asb}}$

best to plot a few points in one of the nasal quadrants and determine where they lie. In this way, a decision to choose another stimulus can be made without a great expenditure of time.

A fundamental understanding of the relative roles that target luminance and target area play in determining total target stimulus is important to choosing the target. To begin, a discussion of base 10 log units is necessary. A number that is one log unit greater than another is that number which is ten times the other. For example, 100 is one log unit greater than 10. Similarly, 10 is one log unit less than 100. However, a number that is one-half a log unit greater than another is that number which is 3.15 times the other. For example, 31.5 is one-half a log unit greater than 10. Obviously, there is a nonlinear relationship between a set of numbers and their logarithms. That is because they are defined as follows:

$$.1 \text{ log unit } = {}^1/_{10} \text{ log unit } = 10^{1/10} = 1.25$$
$$.5 \text{ log unit } = {}^1/_2 \text{ log unit } = 10^{1/2} = 3.15$$
$$.6 \text{ log unit } = {}^6/_{10} \text{ log unit } = 10^{6/10} = 4.$$
$$1 \text{ log unit } = {}^1/_1 \text{ log unit } = 10^{1/1} = 10.$$
$$2 \text{ log units } = {}^2/_1 \text{ log unit } = 10^{2/1} = 100$$
$$4 \text{ log units } = {}^4/_1 \text{ log unit } = 10^{4/1} = 10,000$$

They are exponential powers and roots of 10.

These logarithms are important to perimetry because Goldmann determined that two isopters of the same radius could be found with different stimuli so long as the area of the target increased as its luminance decreased. In fact, he thought that a .5 log unit increase in luminance (3.15×) had to be offset by a .6 log unit decrease in area (1/4×) for the total target stimulus to be equivalent. Although some discrepancy with this ratio has been found since Goldmann's calculations, especially for peripheral isopters, it is basically correct.

As a result of Goldmann's concepts, his kinetic perimeter was designed with target areas that can be varied in multiples of four (.6 log unit). The luminance values can be varied in multiples of 3.15 (.5 log unit), as well as in multiples of 1.25 (.1 log unit).

A Haag-Streit Goldmann kinetic perimeter has three levers: one for target area, and two for luminance. (The perimeters with static capabilities have a third luminance lever, which should remain on 1.00× during kinetic use). The target area notations are in Roman numerals, 0, I, II, III, IV, V, which represent 1/16 mm², 1/4 mm², 1 mm², 4 mm², 16 mm², and 64 mm² respectively (4× multiples of each other). The major target luminance lever uses Arabic numerals, 1, 2, 3, 4, which represent 31.5 asb, 100 asb, 315 asb, and 1000 asb respectively (3.15× multiples of each other), as long as the second luminance lever is set on small letter e, which allows 1.00× or 100% of light to pass through. If this second lever is moved to d, c, b, or a, the total luminance is decreased to .8×, .63×, .5× or .4× respectively, representing .1 log unit differences (1.25× multiples of each other). Both target luminance levers are thereby used to reduce the total projected intensity of the perimeter's bulb (1000 asb) by the percentage specified, but expressed as a decimal. In fact, the Arabic 1, 2, 3, 4 filters transmit .0315×, .100×, .315× and 1.00× of the 1000 asb bulb respectively; that is, 31.5 asb (.0315 × 1000 = 31.5), 100 asb, 315 asb, and 1000 asb as previously described. When the e filter is in place, this is the exact luminance of the target because the e filter allows complete transmission of light (1.00×).

If the Arabic lever is set on 4 (1.00× transmission) and the letter lever on e (1.00× transmission), then the target has a luminance of 1000 asb (1.00 × 1.00 × 1000 asb). If the Arabic lever is set on 4 (1.00× transmission) and the letter lever on c (.63 × transmission), then the target has a luminance of 630 asb (1.00 × .63 × 1000 asb).

Mastery of this mathematical system of expressing change

in total target stimulus by altering its area and its luminance will significantly enhance the art of perimetry. Coupled with the proper method of target presentation, a clinically reliable record of the patient's visual field can be obtained each time the test is performed.

ROUTINE STATIC PERIMETRY (THRESHOLD PROFILE PERIMETRY)

Special Considerations and Filter Characteristics

In situations in which isopter perimetry does not provide sufficient diagnostic information, threshold static perimetry is necessary. This test is usually performed only within the central 30 degrees and with the spectacle correction in place.

Because the central hole in the Goldmann perimeter for the perimetrist's telescope is approximately 2 degrees in diameter, the area near fixation must be tested at a location in the dome that is 5 degrees from the center of the hole. A special attachment is provided to project a pericentral fixation target there. In this way, the patient fixates with his perimacular area so that the threshold at every degree of the fovea and macula can be measured without interference.

Another peculiarity of the Goldmann perimeter is that it has a third target luminance filter for static perimetry. As previously alluded to the lowest Arabic luminance filter setting (1) combined with the lowest letter luminance filter setting (a) yields 12.5 asb of light. However, foveal sensitivity at 31.5 asb of background illumination may be as much as 1 log unit less than this (.1 × 12.5 asb = 1.25 asb). To obtain this low level of light, another luminance filter is provided that affects the transmission of target intensity by either no reduction (1.00×), a 2-log unit reduction (.01×), or a 4-log unit reduction (.0001×). The notation for .01× is a single bar (−). The notation for .0001 × is a double bar (=).

While performing routine visual field testing, this third luminance lever should remain on 1.00×. Otherwise, the target luminance will not be great enough for testing, because the most light that can be transmitted with the single bar filter (—) in place is 10 asb (.01 × 1000 asb), less stimulus than is required for kinetic work. However, in threshold static perimetry there is frequent need for intensities that are this low and lower. To obtain them, combinations of the single bar filter (.01×), the 3 (.315×) and 4 (1.00×) Arabic filters, and the complete range of letter filters are required. For example, to obtain 1.25 asb of luminance, the filter notations should be set at 3̄a (.315 × .4 × .01 × 1000 asb = 1.25 asb).To obtain 10 asb of luminance, 4̄e should be used (1.00 × 1.00 × .01 × 1000 asb = 10 asb). At 12.5 asb and above, only the Arabic and letter filters need to be manipulated to change the target luminance while the third luminance filter remains on 1.00×.

Although combinations of three luminance levers can achieve all necessary levels of light stimulus, they are cumbersome to maneuver while simultaneously attempting to hold the target steady and move quickly from location to location. Nonetheless, adequate static perimetry can be done with the Goldmann machine by an experienced perimetrist.

Target Choices

Throughout Goldmann threshold static perimetry, the target size should remain constant at 1/4 mm² (I). The foveal threshold should be determined first by setting the luminance at 1.25 asb and increasing it in steps of .1 log unit at a time, with .5-second exposure at each level, until the patient

Chart 5-4.   Routine Static Perimetry

1. Keep the target area constant.
2. Change the target luminance in 1.25× multiples.
3. Expose the stimulus for .5 second.
4. Use a pericentral fixation target.
5. Explore four meridians routinely (45, 135, 225, and 315 degrees) and check any dips in them by using circular static perimetry.

responds. At this test point (0 degrees), as well as all others, it is best to obtain two negative answers at two successive luminances before accepting a positive response. This requirement is necessary to guarantee that testing was begun at a subthreshold level. Unless this is done, the actual threshold cannot be measured before dazzling the patient with a suprathreshold target. This excessive amount of stimulation causes local adaptation to dimmer stimuli, a phenomenon that will negatively influence the reliability of the results.

Finding the right subthreshold target at each location on the meridian is best done by first decreasing the luminance of the target that was just seen at the previous test point by .4 log units. Because the normal threshold profile gradually slopes toward brighter luminances as it moves from 0 to 30 degrees, this is an efficient method of dimming the stimulus sufficiently that the obligatory number of negative responses to light will be obtained before the threshold is identified. In abnormal areas of meridians where large dips of sensitivity are found, fulfilling these test criteria may be more difficult. In these situations, a good general rule for dimming the target before proceeding to the next test point is as follows: Count the number of .1 log units from the top of the dip at which the previous point's target had to be brightened before it was perceived. Add this number to .4 log units and dim the stimulus for the next location to be tested by that sum (Fig. 5-10). Although there is no perfect formula for choosing the proper luminance from which to begin the examination of each location, the test will be expedited by using a consistent approach such as this.

Presentation Patterns

After testing the sensitivity to light at 0 degrees, four meridians should be routinely explored: 45, 135, 225, and 315 degrees. Each radius degree should be examined from 0 to 20 degrees, and every second degree, from 20 to 30

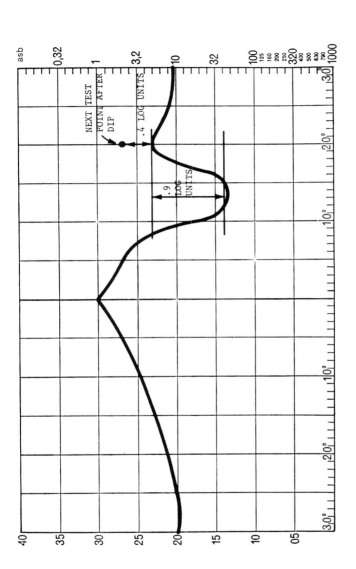

Fig. 5-10. Determination of initial subthreshold target intensity for static threshold perimetry.

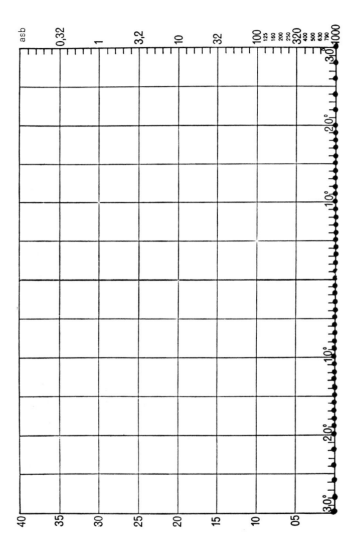

Fig. 5-11. Radial static perimetry check points.

degrees, using .5-second target exposure with a three-second pause between them (Fig. 5-11). The meridional examination need not be limited to the four standard meridians, but should be expanded to include any other meridian in which there is reason to suspect a defect. The meridians at 45, 135, 225, and 315 degrees have been selected for testing because at least a portion of most scotomas seem to be found at these locations.

Once the examination has reached 3 degrees radius on all meridians, the patient's fixation should be directed to the center of the dome and the pericentral fixation target should be removed. Before doing this, however, the variation of each individual's threshold sensitivity should be measured. This is done by selecting a segment of the inferior nasal meridian at a radius of approximately 2 to 5 degrees and testing each degree twice. The magnitude of this variation is crucial to the interpretation of the significance of early glaucomatous defects.

The final phase of threshold static perimetry, the circular examination, should be performed wherever dips on the meridional profile are found that suggest glaucoma. The same target area and choice of luminance are used as in meridional static perimetry, but the test proceeds around a portion or all of one concentric circle. The circular approach identifies the full circumference of the defect.

Static perimetry might be used for the workup of a glaucoma patient in two clinical situations: (1) to examine patients whose optic discs are suspicious of disease but who demonstrate no scotoma on kinetic testing; (2) to explore more fully the visual field of a known glaucoma patient, which can establish a detailed baseline with which to compare the results of subsequent perimetry. Both circumstances are appropriate indications for this technique, which should be employed whenever any doubt exists about the real status of a patient's visual field.

Chapter 6

STEREOSCOPIC EVALUATION OF
THE OPTIC CUP

Just as the ophthalmoscope is relatively limited in its ability to provide enough magnification to produce high resolution of retinal structure, it is also limited for evaluating the optic disc. To determine whether early glaucomatous changes exist or minimal progression has occurred in comparison with previous examinations of the optic cup, only a stereoscopic view with a slit lamp will suffice. With this instrument, either a Goldmann fundus contact lens or a Hruby lens will be necessary. The latter has the advantage of not clouding the corneal epithelium, which allows one to take clear post-examination photographs of the optic nerve head if they are desired.

It is the evaluation of the three-dimensional structure of the optic cup, not its color, surface orifice, or major vessel location, that is essential to deciding correctly whether and where the nerve head is glaucomatous. The basic patterns of normal and abnormal discs have already been described in the section on diagnosis and therapy and are referred to here wherever appropriate. However, this chapter primarily emphasizes how one goes about seeing the necessary details.

A full-height, narrow, slit beam should be used and kept slightly off center most of the time. During the examination, the position of the beam must be changed frequently in order to highlight all portions of the disc.

THE NORMAL CUP

At the start of the evaluation procedure, a determination should be made whether the lamina can be seen deep in the cup. Then the slope of the superior contour of the cup should be examined, especially its superior temporal aspect. Evaluate the steepness of the wall of the cup as it descends from the surface of the nerve head to the lamina (if it is visible) or to the top of the central prelaminar tissue. One of three basic patterns is likely: heavily slanted but straight, nearly perpendicular, or gradually curving (Fig. 6-1), so that the superior half of the cup geometrically resembles half of the inside of a cone, a cylinder, or a hemisphere, respectively. The slope of the inferior temporal contour of the cup should be inspected to determine its configuration as well.

Because nerve rim overhangs occur in at least 50% of normal subjects, they are not helpful and are often confusing in the differentiation of glaucomatous change. Although undermining may occur as glaucomatous atrophy progresses, other, more consistently reliable signs of this disease can and should be used for evaluation. In fact, since it is not possible to see very far under rim overhangs, it is more helpful to assume that such an edge is really a perpendicular wall from the top to the bottom of the cup (Fig. 6-2).

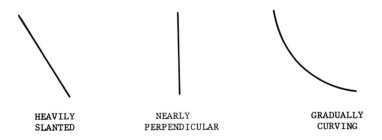

| HEAVILY SLANTED | NEARLY PERPENDICULAR | GRADUALLY CURVING |

Fig. 6-1.   Cup slope patterns.

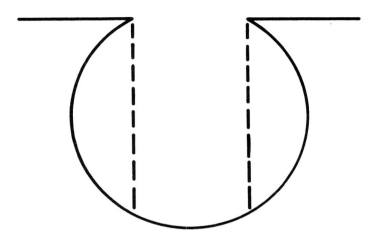

Fig. 6-2. Assumption of cup wall perpendicularity instead of overhang.

The shapes of the superior and inferior areas of the cup on the *temporal* side are emphasized because overhangs in normal discs usually occur nasally. With the evaluation scheme presented here, these overhangs would be treated as perpendicular edges, which would tend to minimize the differences in structure that exist among optic cups if too much attention were paid to their nasal side.

One should be able to classify most optic cups into one of nine geometric shapes, by combining the results of evaluation of their top and bottom halves respectively: cone-cone, cylinder-cylinder, hemisphere-hemisphere (or simply cone, cylinder, or hemisphere), cone-cylinder, cylinder-cone, hemisphere-cone, cone-hemisphere, cylinder-hemisphere, and hemisphere-cylinder. Of all these types, cone-shaped cups are *least* likely to reach the lamina.

THE GLAUCOMATOUS CUP

The foregoing categories are intended for the classification of normal cups only. Furthermore, there is little likelihood that one of those shapes can be altered with time and maintain a configuration identical to its former self. Nevertheless, a glaucomatous cup may occasionally mimic a normal cup. Under these circumstances, the two most valuable aids in differentiating between normal and glaucomatous discs are the presence of cup asymmetry between the patient's two eyes and the appearance of rarefied tissue anywhere around the perimeter of the cup.

Theoretically, the nutrition of the optic disc is compromised, which leads to thinning out of the nerve tissue and the formation of a mosaic of irregularly placed semitransparent filmy patches interposed among normal areas just beneath the lining of the cup. This is particularly evident at the bases of cups that do not reach the lamina before they become glaucomatous, such as those that are cone-shaped, and it is even more obvious when one can compare this rarefaction with the more solid appearing normal nerve tissue on the other side. As this architectural derangement progresses, the former surface of the cup may still be visible, but without any obvious prelaminar support beneath it. That is, a veil of tissue seems to be suspended in the center of the nerve head, as if hanging in space without a firm foundation. If a small blood vessel is still present in this tissue, it will be more easily noticeable.

When the surface veil finally disappears, the formerly cone-shaped cup may be transformed into a cylinder that is ophthalmoscopically indistinguishable from the normal cylinder. Of course, in the vast majority of cases, if the other eye's optic nerve head is normal and has a cone-shaped cup, this asymmetry is strongly suggestive of the presence of glaucoma in the eye with the cylinder-shaped cup. The only other way of making this differentiation is to find areas of rarefaction of the nerve tissue around the cup's borders. In most glaucomatous discs, it is possible to see this change by using the magnification and stereopsis available with the slit lamp.

In fact, only in cups that do not reach the lamina prior to the onset of glaucoma is there sufficient prelaminar tissue in which to find this patchy filminess. Once the loss of this tissue is complete, further deepening of the cup does not occur until very late in the disease. Instead, these cups, as well as those that did not normally reach the lamina, undergo rarefaction and subsequent atrophy around their edges.

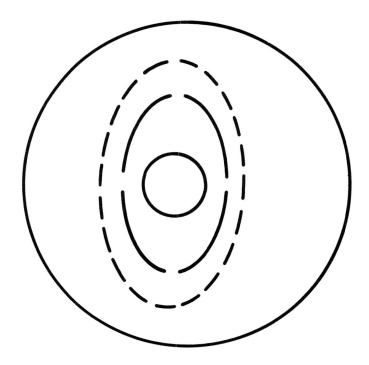

Fig. 6-3. Cycles of concentrically expanding vertically oval glaucomatous cups.

The same semitransparent changes can be seen around the borders of the cup, down its walls, and on the nerve head surface. The atrophy that follows enlarges the cup diameter at its depth as well as at its orifice. Thus, a pattern of vertically oriented, concentrically expanding ellipses of destruction occurs in cycles of rarefaction alternating with atrophy followed again by rarefaction of the "new" cup edge (Fig. 6-3).

Because the cup is normally located somewhat on the temporal side of the disc, this process of predominantly vertical atrophy, coupled with a less noticeable but definite horizontal expansion of the cup, first causes the inferior temporal and superior temporal cup rims to disappear, though not usually at the same time. After the atrophy has reached those margins, the temporal rim becomes smaller and eventually disappears. While this is happening, the nasal rim gradually narrows but remains present, in part, until the last.

The later stages of optic disc atrophy can be seen with the ophthalmoscope alone, especially after the inferior or superior poles of the cup have extended to the edge of the retina. However, the value of a stereo view with the slit lamp lies in its ability to focus on the subtle rarefied areas of the disc that precede more obvious atrophy, that indicate that the glaucomatous process is still unchecked, and that may not alter the cup/disc ratio. Furthermore, paying careful attention to the area of the disc immediately surrounding the cup on all sides (which is possible only with this degree of stereoscopic magnification) is essential to identifying nerve head damage in the earliest phases of disease.

The possibility that glaucomatous cups that have not excavated to the margin of the disc may be confused with normal cups does not significantly detract from the value of a three-dimensional geometric classification for normal cups; rather, it emphasizes the necessity to look at them closely with the slit lamp. In fact, this system is particularly useful because it provides a simple method of chart notation (Fig. 6-4)

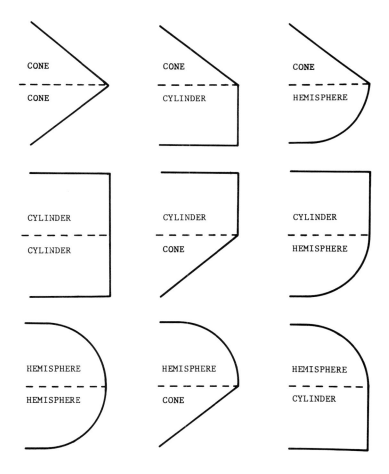

Fig. 6-4. Chart notations for normal cup halves.

without the need for a photograph while giving more detail than a cup/disc ratio alone. This enhances comparison with previous examination records and directs the attention of the ophthalmologist to the subtle filmy change that is a basic component of glaucomatous atrophy.

SPECIAL CONSIDERATIONS

There are two possible areas of confusion in the disc examination. The first is that of mistaking a blood vessel that has the normal structural "strength" to stand out from the bottom of the cup without obvious support for one that is in a similar position but whose foundation has disappeared as a result of glaucoma. This is a difficult distinction, but it can be approached by determining, with the slit lamp on high magnification, whether the walls of the vessel in question can be differentiated clearly from its blood column. If not, then one can decide arbitrarily that the tissue support of the vessel has probably atrophied, because under normal conditions it would be too thin to stand freely. In such cases, some residual rarefied portion of the nerve usually is visible nearby to suggest the presence of disease.

Another area of possible confusion is that of mistaking a peripapillary scleral halo for residual nerve rim. This would erroneously lead to a conclusion that the cup has not yet excavated the disc margin. One way of avoiding this pitfall is to learn to distinguish the starker whiteness of adjacent sclera or scleral lip over a cup from the pallor of diseased nerve tissue. Another useful method would involve finding a portion of the disc border (usually nasally) where one can definitely determine the junction of nerve head with sclera or retina, and following that arc around to the area in question. If a relatively ragged curve or a horizontal edge leads to the location of questionable disc-retinal transition or scleral-retinal junction, then one can assume that it is actually the scleral-retinal junction that is being seen (Fig. 6-5).

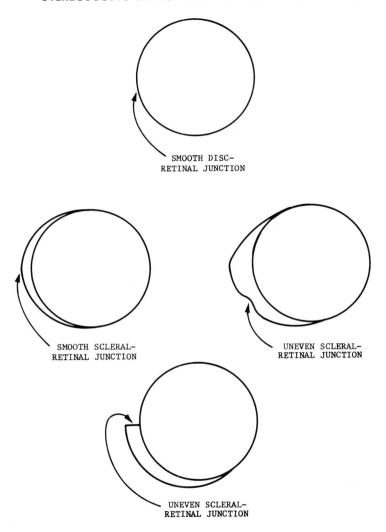

Fig. 6-5. Patterns of disc-retinal and scleral-retinal transition.

Even after becoming completely familiar with all aspects of optic cup evaluation, many subtle disc features will be found that will give rise to questions with regard to their significance. Because the techniques for accurate optic nerve head analysis are still evolving, it is useful to compare the results of optic disc examination closely with those of quantitative perimetry. With this approach, one can gain increased confidence in the results of disc evaluation.

Section III

Background on Glaucoma

Chapter 7

THE ETIOLOGY OF GLAUCOMA: PAST, PRESENT, AND FUTURE THEORIES

THE COLLECTION OF CLUES

Prior to the mid-1930's, the differentiation of open-angle versus angle-closure glaucoma hardly existed because of the prevailing idea that all cases of glaucoma had one cause—that is, they were all caused by iridial or synechial blocks of the trabecular meshwork. The period starting with the year 1938, in fact, marks the beginning of the "present" epoch in the etiology of glaucoma.

The "past" might well begin with MacKenzie in 1835, who was the first to establish that glaucoma was a disease of elevated intraocular pressure. However, not until the invention of the ophthalmoscope, which permitted a view of the cupped glaucomatous disc, did this definition become widely accepted.

As proposed by von Graefe[1] in 1854 (among others), this "hypertension" was caused by hypersecretion of aqueous. However, Bowman[2] in 1862 thought that an excessively large lens might be responsible for creating an anatomic block to aqueous outflow, which, in turn, made the intraocular pressure rise. Knies[3] in 1876 and Weber[4] in 1877, working independently on the anatomic examination of enucleated eyes, added support to the idea of restricted outflow by finding peripheral synechiae in the chamber angle, which they concluded were the source of obstruction. Priestly Smith,[5] in 1887, renewed interest in the lens as the major obstruction to aqueous outflow in all cases of glaucoma by suggesting that the continual increase in lens size that occurs with age was at fault. He also believed that most glaucomatous eyes possessed a shallow anterior chamber, an idea that has maintained popularity as late as 1936 and even beyond.[6]

As more investigators became involved, bits and pieces of this complex puzzle began to fall into place. Gronholm[7] in 1910 reported that intraocular pressure elevated in response to the dark. In 1920, Seidel suggested the concept of relative pupillary block, and Curran[8] emphasized its significance. Seidel,[9] in 1928, suggested that mydriasis caused the iris to bunch in the angle, accompanied by a reduction in aqueous outflow.

"Peripheral anterior synechiae were widely believed to be the cause of most cases of glaucoma, a belief based on their constant occurrence found (histologically) in eyes enucleated for absolute glaucoma, but with the advent of gonioscopy doubts began to be cast on the theory."[10] Salzmann,[11] in 1914, using gonioscopy, showed that peripheral anterior synechiae were not present in many early cases of glaucoma and, therefore, could not be the sole reason for its development.

At that time, glaucoma was classified into categories such as acute, subacute, chronic, compensated, noncompensated, congestive, or noncongestive, based on empirical observations and symptoms rather than etiology. Although Raeder[12] in 1923 had differentiated between deep-chamber and shallow-chamber glaucoma, it was not until 1938 when Barkan[13] clearly established the fact that primary glaucoma was not due to a single defect. His description of wide-angle and narrow-angle categories provided the basis for the present day approach to classification of this disease.

quantification of autonomic effector substances in the control of intraocular pressure.

The biochemical effect of ascorbic acid on intraocular pressure was reported by Linner[42] in 1964. Both topical application and systemic administration of ascorbic acid resulted in a slight fall in tension. According to Linner, if we can assume that the outflow channels are affected, a possible explanation for the pressure reduction might be a de-polymerizing effect on the mucopolysaccharides in the trabecular meshwork. Perhaps the normal relatively high level of ascorbic acid in the aqueous is necessary to maintain the patency of the outflow channels. It is well-known that prolonged administration of ACTH leads to impoverishment of ascorbic acid in the adrenal cortex. In addition, Cucco and Montanari[43] in 1951 found a reduction in the depolymerizing activity of aqueous after similar prolonged administration of ACTH, which may be due to similar ascorbic acid depletion. Therefore, an equilibrium may exist between steroids and ascorbic acid such that a normal aqueous depolymerizing activity maintains a proper mucopolysaccharide status. An imbalance of this biochemical system may provide another basis for an increase in intraocular pressure.

In general, the idea that an anatomic block to outflow exists in open-angle glaucoma may be out of date. The confusion arising from the long-standing failure to differentiate between eyes with narrow angles and those with open angles may still cloud the issue, owing to persistence of the idea that some unidentified anatomic block must indeed be the cause of open-angle glaucoma because a structural abnormality is responsible for angle-closure.

THE EVOLUTION OF ANGLE-CLOSURE GLAUCOMA

Some comments on the etiology of angle-closure glaucoma are appropriate. The main reason for the increased intraocular pressure in this disease is occlusion of the trabecular meshwork by the iris. However, of major concern in this type of primary glaucoma is the constellation of various factors that make the eye susceptible to this event and the exact manner in which it happens.

The real understanding of the etiology of angle-closure glaucoma dates back only to Barkan's description in 1938. As has been described, many authors had already collectively discovered the important etiologic elements of angle-closure glaucoma. The only thing left to explain was how these elements interacted. The main predisposing structural problem is that the anterior chamber is narrow, the iris is more convex than usual and, as a result, its peripheral portion comes into close proximity with the trabecular meshwork. This situation might be called physiologic iris bombé. Occasionally, a flatter iris is found along with a prominent last roll at its base, a configuration that was called a plateau type of iris by Shaffer[44] in 1960.

Rosengren[45] in 1953 demonstrated that the degree of shallowness of the anterior chamber is not the result of an acute episode of angle-closure glaucoma and is not increased during an attack, but is a constant dimension of the eye. The only variation in this depth seems to be an increase in the shallowness that occurs with increasing age, owing to an increase in growth of the lens as had already been described by Priestly Smith. Some anterior displacement of the lens in the eye may occur during an attack, but there is no proof of such a change.

As previously mentioned, the degree of tautness of the iris diaphragm appears to be an important variable. Marr[46] in 1947 and Haas[47] in 1948 showed that the strong miotic di-isopropyl fluorophosphate (DFP), which might be expected to tighten the iris diaphragm and pull it away from the trabeculum, can precipitate an episode of angle-closure glaucoma if other conditions are met. The cause of this may be iris or ciliary body vascular congestion, an alteration in the structure and position of the ciliary muscle, or an increase in pupillary block produced by the miosis. According to Redmond Smith,[48] "an important factor would be the relationship between the degree of miosis obtained compared with the degree of tautening of the iris diaphragm which results. If the total area of the diaphragm were sufficiently large to allow pinpoint (miosis) without necessarily causing tautening and flattening of the entire diaphragm, such an eye would be more likely to succumb to DFP miosis than one in which, due to a slightly 'smaller' iris, extreme miosis produced an iris diaphragm as taut as a 'drum'."

As pointed out by Chandler[49] in 1952, the iris around the pupil may have so much contact with the lens that an abnormal resistance to aqueous flow through the pupil develops. The extent of this pupillary block, combined with the concurrent physiologic iris bombé, may change as the pupil size varies while simultaneous alterations occur in the flaccidity of the iris diaphragm. Thus, the amount of forward movement of the peripheral part of the iris has many causes—pupillary block, flaccidity of the diaphragm, and the flow rate of aqueous. Posner[50] in 1952 even suggested that the base of the iris might be sucked toward the meshwork owing to an abrupt lowering of pressure in the canal of Schlemm. A rapid surge in the formation of aqueous might also contribute to the problem, as suggested by the fact that the water drinking test is frequently positive in eyes with angle-closure glaucoma.[51]

MULTIPLE CAUSES

Clearly, the causes of angle-closure glaucoma are multifactorial. These factors have been well-described and have pointed the way toward successful care of patients with this problem.

Recent research suggests that open-angle glaucoma might also be a multifactorial disease. By way of comparison, human blood pressure depends on a variety of mechanisms for control. There is no apparent reason why intraocular pressure cannot qualify for a similar type of regulation. Understanding the interrelationships of the mechanisms that have been postulated in the etiology of open-angle glaucoma would seem to be the logical goal for future research.

Electron microscopic studies by Tripathi[52,53] in 1968 and 1972 and Inomata et al.[54] in 1972, have begun to point in this direction. Their work suggests that the outflow of aqueous through the endothelium that lines the inner wall of Schlemm's canal depends on a physiologically *and* anatomically active process of endothelial vacuolization. That is, vacuoles form in these cells and eventually rupture into the canal, perhaps under the influence of pinocytosis as well as hydrostatic pressure. By doing so, they provide a temporary through-and-through pathway for the flow of fluid. Later, the cytoplasm of the cell fills the base of the ruptured vacuole and occludes the channel at its base.

The mathematical breakdown of aqueous production into components of active secretion and passive ultrafiltration (pseudofacility) was initially described by Barany[55] in 1963 and later elaborated upon by Goldmann[56] in 1968. Through the efforts of Kupfer, Ross, Gaasterland, et al.[57-60] between 1971 and 1975, a precise analysis of the effects of a variety of drugs on these properties as well as on true outflow facility has been achieved. This work was best summarized by Kupfer[61] in 1973, who drew attention to the finding that epinephrine greatly decreases pseudofacility and flow in young subjects but not in older ones. On the other hand, pilocarpine causes an increase in pseudofacility and a decrease in flow. These results open up the entire subject of autonomic regulation of intraocular pressure by suggesting that sympathomimetics may have a minimal influence on inflow in contrast to that of parasympathomimetics, especially in older people, a situation contrary to previous impressions.

The individual roles of alpha versus beta sympathetic stimulation in the eyes of rabbits have been increasingly separated from each other as an outgrowth of further work of

Barany[62] and Langham et al.[63-65] This has been made possible by the relatively recent availability of specific inhibitors of adrenergic receptors. Although both alpha and beta stimulation decrease intraocular pressure in these animals, alpha stimulation appears to be most effective. Furthermore, this pressure regulation seems to depend on vasomotor responses in the anterior uveal circulation, where the aqueous drains. Thus, increased attention is being directed to uveal-scleral outflow, whose pathologic alterations may be a significant event in the development of glaucoma.

The entire subject of autonomic control of intraocular pressure requires further quantification in order to clarify some of the discrepancies of drug effects that have been reported among animals and humans[66-67] and to make the results more clinically applicable. To do so, future research into the underlying abnormalities in open-angle glaucoma will depend even more heavily on the development and application of refined laboratory microtechniques. Such efforts in the areas of cellular biochemistry, block specific pharmacology, electron microscopy, and even microsurgery, may soon bring this whole field into perspective.

REFERENCES

1. von Graefe, A.: Vorläufige Notiz über das Wesen des Glaucoma. Arch. Ophthalmol. 1:371-382, 1854.
2. Bowman, W.: On glaucomatous affections and their treatment by iridectomy. Br. Med. J. 2:377-382, 1862.
3. Knies, M.: Ueber des Glaucom. Albrecht von Graefes Arch. Ophthalmol. 22:163-202, 1876
4. Weber, A.: Die Ursache des Glaucoms. Albrecht von Graefes Arch. Ophthalmol. 23:1-91, 1877.
5. Smith, P.: On the shallow anterior chamber of primary glaucoma. Ophthal. Rev. 6:191-198, 1887.
6. Gradle, H. S.: Glaucoma. In C. Berens (ed.): The Eye and Its Disease. Philadelphia, W. B. Saunders, 1936. pp. 699-732.
7. Gronholm, V.: Untersuchungen über den Einfluss der Pupillenweite, der Accomodation und der Convergenz auf die Tension glaucomatöser und normaler Augen. Arch. Augenheilk. 67:136-182, 1910.

8. Curran, E. J.: A new operation for glaucoma involving a new principle in the aetiology and treatment of chronic primary glaucoma. Arch. Ophthalmol. 49:131-155, 1920.

9. Seidel, E.: Zur Methodik der klinischen glaukomforschung. Albrecht von Graefes Arch. Ophthalmol. 119:15-21, 1927.

10. Smith, R. J. H.: *Clinical Glaucoma.* London, Cassell and Company Ltd., 1965. p. 41.

11. Salzmann, M.: Die Ophthalmoskopie der Kammerbucht. Z. Augenheilk. 31:1-19, 1914.

12. Raeder, J. G.: Untersuchungen über die Lage und Dicke der Linse im menschlichen Auge bei physiologischen und pathologischen Zuständen, nach einer neuen Methode gemessen. Albrecht von Graefes Arch. Ophthalmol. 112:29-63, 1923.

13. Barkan, O.: Glaucoma: classification, causes, and surgical control. Am. J. Ophthalmol. 21:1099-1117, 1938.

14. Grant, W. M.: Tonographic method for measuring the facility and rate of aqueous flow in human eyes. Arch. Ophthalmol. 44:204-214, 1950.

15. Goldmann, von H.: Das Minutenvolumen der menschlichen Vorderkammer bei Normalen und bei Fällen von primärem Glaukom. Ophthalmologica, 120:150-156, 1950.

16. Kronfeld, P. C., McGarry, H. I., and Smith, H. E.: Gonioscopic studies on the canal of Schlemm. Am. J. Ophthalmol. 25:1163-1173, 1942.

17. Kronfeld, P.: Further gonioscopic studies on the canal of Schlemm. Arch. Ophthalmol. 41:393-405, 1949.

18. Henderson, T.: Anatomical factors bearing on the pathogenesis of glaucoma. Ophthal. Rec. 17:534-536, 1908.

19. Anderson, D. R.: Pathology of the glaucomas. Br. J. Ophthalmol. 56:146-157, 1972.

20. Teng, C. C., Paton, R. T., and Katzin, H. M.: Primary degeneration in the vicinity of the chamber angle. Am. J. Ophthalmol. 40:619-631, 1955.

21. Theobald, G. D.: Further studies on the canal of Schlemm: Its anastomoses and anatomic relations. Am. J. Ophthalmol. 39 (4/Part 2):65-89, 1955.

22. Kornzweig, A. L., Feldstein, M. D., and Schneider, J.: Pathology of the angle of the anterior chamber in primary glaucoma. Am. J. Ophthalmol. 46:311-327, 1958.

23. Flocks, M.: The pathology of the trabecular meshwork in primary open-angle glaucoma. Am. J. Ophthalmol. 47:519-536, 1959.

24. Levinsohn, G.: Beitrag zur pathologischen Anatomie und Pathogenese des Glaucoms. Arch. Augenheilk. 62:131-154, 1909.

25. Francois, J.: La gonioscopie dans le glaucome primitif. Ann. Ocul. 181:399-409, 1948.

26. Sugar, H. S.: Concerning the chamber angle. I. Gonioscopy. Am. J. Ophthalmol. 23:853-866, 1940.

27. Barkan, O.: Primary glaucoma: pathogenesis and classification. Am. J. Ophthalmol. 37:724-744, 1954.

28. Barany, E. H.: Physiologic and pharmacologic factors influencing the resistance to aqueous flow. *In* Glaucoma: Transactions of the First

Conference, Princeton, December 5-7, 1955. New York, Josiah Macy, Jr. Foundation, 1956. pp. 123-221.
29. Brini, M. A.: Mise en évidence, à l'aide de techniques histochimgues, d'une substance sensible à l'hyaluronidase dans le trabéculum de l'oeil humain. Bull. Soc. Ophthalmol. Fr. 1956:256-264, 1956.
30. Zimmerman, L. E.: Demonstration of hyaluronidase-sensitive acid mucopolysaccharide. Am. J. Ophthalmol. 44:1-4, 1957.
31. Meyer, K.: The biological significance of hyaluronic acid and hyaluronidase. Physiol. Rev. 27:335-359, 1947.
32. Thomson, A.: The filtration angle. Ophthalmoscope. 9:470-472, 1911.
33. Fortin, E. P.: La contraction de muscle ciliare ouvre le canal de Schlemm. Semana Med. 36:209-213, 1929.
34. Flocks, M., and Zweng, H. C.: Studies on the mode of action of pilocarpine on aqueous outflow. Am. J. Ophthalmol. 44(5/part II): 380-388, 1957.
35. Christensen, R. E., and Pearce, I.: Homatropine hydrobromide. Arch. Ophthalmol. 70:376-380, 1963.
36. Smith, R. J. H.: Clinical Glaucoma. London, Cassell and Co. Ltd., 1965. p. 45.
37. Friedenwald, J. S.: Circulation of the aqueous. V. Mechanism of Schlemm's canal. Arch. Ophthalmol. 16:65-77, 1936.
38. Ashton, N., and Smith, R.: Anatomical study of Schlemm's canal and aqueous veins by means of neoprene casts. III. Arteriol relations of Schlemm's canal. Br. J. Ophthalmol. 37:577-586, 1953.
39. Duke-Elder, W. S.: Textbook of Ophthalmology. London, Kempton, 1940. p. 3357.
40. Feeney, L., and Wissig, L.: Outflow studies using an electron dense tracer. Trans. Am. Acad. Ophthalmol. Otolaryngol. 70:791-798, 1967.
41. Sears, M. L., and Barany, E. H.: Outflow resistance and adrenergic mechanisms. Arch. Ophthalmol. 64:839-848, 1960.
42. Linner, E.: Corticosteroid hormones, ascorbic acid and intraocular pressure. Acta Ophthalmol. 42:932-933, 1964.
43. Cucco, G., and Montanari, L.: Influence exercée par certaines hormones (ACTH, Dopa, ACE) sur la teneur en hyaluronidase de l'humeur aqueuse. Ann. Ocul. 184:550-551, 1951.
44. Shaffer, R. N.: Gonioscopy, ophthalmoscopy, and perimetry. Trans. Am. Acad. Ophthalmol. Otolaryngol. 64:112-127, 1960.
45. Rosengren, B.: The etiology of acute glaucoma. Am. J. Ophthalmol. 36:488-492, 1953.
46. Marr, W. G.: The clinical use of di-isopropyl fluorophosphate (DFP) in chronic glaucoma. Am. J. Ophthalmol. 30:1423-1428, 1947.
47. Haas, J. S.: Response to DFP. Am. J. Ophthalmol. 31:227-228, 1948.
48. Smith, R. J. H.: Clinical Glaucoma. London, Cassell and Co. Ltd., 1965. p. 50.
49. Chandler, P. A.: Narrow-angle glaucoma. Arch. Ophthalmol. 47:695-716, 1952.
50. Posner, A.: Suction on iris as a cause of acute narrow angle glaucoma. Eye Ear Nose Throat Mon. 31:563 (Passim), 1952.

51. Leydhecker, W.: The water-drinking test. Br. J. Ophthalmol. 34:457-479, 1950.
52. Tripathi, R. C.: Aqueous outflow pathway in normal and glaucomatous eyes. Br. J. Ophthalmol. 56:157-174, 1972.
53. ———: Ultrastructure of Schlemm's canal in relation to aqueous outflow. Exp. Eye Res. 7:335-341, 1968.
54. Inomata, H., Bill, A., and Smelser, G. K.: Aqueous humor pathways through the trabecular meshwork and into Schlemm's canal in the Cynomolgus monkey (Macaca irus). Am. J. Ophthalmol. 73:760-789, 1972.
55. Barany, E. H.: A mathematical formulation of intraocular pressure as dependent on secretion, ultrafiltration, bulk outflow, and osmotic reabsorption of fluid. Invest. Ophthalmol. 2:584-590, 1963.
56. Goldmann, H.: On pseudofacility. Bibl. Ophthalmol. 76:1-14, 1968.
57. Kupfer, C., and Ross, K.: Studies of aqueous humor dynamics in man. I. Measurements in young normal subjects. Invest. Ophthalmol. 10:518-522, 1971.
58. Kupfer, C., Gaasterland, D., and Ross, K.: Studies of aqueous humor dynamics in man. II. Measurements in young normal subjects using acetazolamide and L-epinephrine. Invest. Ophthalmol. 10:523-533, 1971.
59. Gaasterland, D., Kupfer, C., Ross, K., and Gabelnick, H. L.: Studies of aqueous humor dynamics in man. III. Measurements in young normal subjects using norepinephrine and isoproterenol. Invest. Ophthalmol. 12:267-279, 1973.
60. Gaasterland., D., Kupfer, C., and Ross, K.: Studies of aqueous humor dynamics in man. IV. Effects of pilocarpine upon measurements in young normal volunteers. Invest. Ophthalmol. 14:848-853, 1975.
61. Kupfer, C.: Clinical significance of pseudofacility. Am. J. Ophthalmol. 75:193-204. 1973.
62. Barany, E. H.: Transient increase in outflow facility after superior cervical ganglionectomy in rabbits. Arch. Ophthalmol. 67:303-311, 1962.
63. Langham, M. E.: The response of the pupil and intraocular pressure of conscious rabbits to adrenergic drugs following unilateral superior cervical ganglionectomy. Exp. Eye Res. 4:381-389, 1965.
64. Langham, M. E., and Diggs, E. M.: Quantitative studies of the ocular response to norepinephrine. Exp. Eye Res. 13:161-171, 1972.
65. Langham, M. E., Simjee, A., and Josephs, S.: The alpha and beta adrenergic responses to epinephrine in the rabbit eye. Exp. Eye Res. 15:75-84, 1973.
66. Kass, M. A., Reid, T. W., Neufeld, A. H., Bausher, L. P., and Sears, M. L.: The effect of d-isoproterenol on intraocular pressure of the rabbit, monkey, and man. Invest. Ophthalmol. 15:113-118, 1976.
67. Chiou, C. Y., and Zimmerman, T. J.: Ocular hypotensive effects of autonomic drugs. Invest. Ophthalmol. 14:416-417, 1975.

GLOSSARY

This Glossary is intended to serve as an easy access dictionary to the specialized scientific language that is used throughout this guidebook. It is oriented toward those readers who do not have an extensive prior knowledge of the eye and

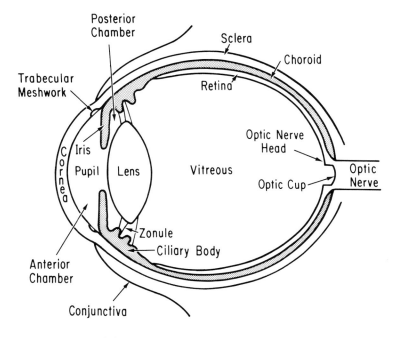

Basic Anatomy of the Eye.

its diseases. The definitions provided here, in a number of instances, have been simplified from their formal meanings in order to convey functional ideas rather than detailed concepts. In particular, this Glossary is directed at the beginner who wishes to acquire familiarity with the terminology that is basic to the language of glaucoma.

accommodation	The focusing of the lens.
acute	Short and perhaps severe.
adrenergic	Sympathetic.
alphachymotrypsin	An enzyme that disintegrates zonules.
anesthetize	To numb.
angle	The angle formed by the junction of the iris and cornea, which is the site of the trabecular meshwork.
angle recession	An abnormal deepening of the anterior chamber angle, usually caused by a tear in the ciliary body.
anterior	In front.
anterior chamber	The space between the iris and the cornea, which normally contains aqueous.
anterior synechiae	Fibrous scars of iridocorneal adhesions, usually located peripherally in the anterior chamber angle.
aphakic	An eye without a crystalline lens.
applanation	The process of flattening a surface.
apostilb (asb)	A measure of luminance. Ten asb equal one millilambert equals 3.183 candle/m^2 (nit).
aqueous	Shortened term for the aqueous humor, which fills the anterior chamber.
aqueous inflow	The production of aqueous by active secretion of the epithelium of the ciliary body and by passive filtration through its blood vessels.
aqueous outflow	The exit of aqueous through the trabecular meshwork, Schlemm's canal and then into the episcleral venous system. Outflow also occurs through uveoscleral pathways that are still incompletely defined.
arachnoid cyst	A cyst of the middle one of the three membranes that cover the brain.

arc	A curved line (e.g., part of a circle).
asb (apostilb)	See apostilb.
astroglia	One type of structural support cells of nerve fibers.
atrophy	Disappearance of tissue.
axoplasmic flow	The movement of metabolic substances through the axon cytoplasm.
bilateral	On both sides.
binocular	Two-eyed.
blepharospasm	Spasm of the eyelids.
blind spot	The portion of the visual field created by the optic nerve head; there are no photo receptors in this area. It is vertically oval (approximately 10 degrees wide and 15 degrees high), and centered at 15 degrees from fixation on the temporal side of the field.
blood staining of cornea	The passage of red blood cells and their breakdown products into the cornea.
brachycardia	Slow heart beat.
bullous keratopathy	A cornea whose subepithelial space is swollen with fluid.
calibrate	To check and correct measurements.
cataract	A lens that is not clear.
capillaries	The smallest blood vessels, either arterial or venous in function.
carbonic anhydrase	The enzyme in the ciliary body that is responsible for the active secretion of aqueous.
carotid	Used to imply the internal carotid artery, one of the major blood vessels supplying the brain.
central vision	Visual acuity of the fovea.
chiasm	The place in the brain where both optic nerves come together and their nasal halves cross.
cholinesterase	An enzyme that destroys acetylcholine.
choroid	The posterior portion of the uvea that separates the retina from the sclera. It provides nutrition to the outer five layers of the retina.
chronic	Long-lasting.

ciliary body

The midportion of the uvea just behind the iris, which lines the inside of the sclera anteriorly. It is functionally responsible for accommodation and aqueous inflow.

coefficient of outflow

See facility of outflow.

conjunctiva

The nearly transparent vessel-containing tissue that covers the anterior sclera and the inside of the lids.

cornea

The clear "watch-glass" that covers the front of the eye.

corneal endothelium

A single layer of cells that lines the inside of the cornea.

corneal epithelium

Multiple layers of cells that cover the outside of the cornea.

corneal lamella

One of the connective tissue sheets of the corneal stroma.

corneal stroma

Multiple sheets of collagen in the center of the cornea, which make up 90% of its thickness.

craniopharyngioma

Benign tumor of the stalk that connects the pituitary gland to the brain; it can press on the chiasm and thereby destroy it.

crystalline lens

See lens.

cyclocryothermy

Freezing of the ciliary body to reduce aqueous production.

cyclodialysis

The artificial separation of ciliary body from sclera.

cycloplegic

A drug that paralyzes the ciliary muscle and dilates the pupil by blocking the parasympathetic receptor sites.

Descemet's membrane

The layer secreted by the corneal endothelium and lying between it and the corneal stroma.

dilator

The radial iris muscle that is primarily responsible for mydriasis.

diurnal

Daily.

edematous

Containing abnormally increased amounts of fluid.

endophthalmitis

Infection of the inside of the eye.

end plate

The junction between a nerve fiber and a muscle fiber.

episcleral veins	The small veins on the surface of the sclera that collect aqueous from Schlemm's canal as well as blood from the anterior superficial portions of the eye.
epithelioid cell	A macrophage that resembles an epithelial cell.
facility of outflow	A measurement of the volume of aqueous that leaves the eye each minute per mm Hg of intraocular pressure (the C value).
fibrin	A product of fibrinogen and thrombin of the blood; forms the basis of scar tissue.
filtering procedure	An operation for the release of aqueous into the subtenon or subconjunctival space by fistulization through the sclera.
fixation	Used to indicate the spot(s) on which a person fixes his gaze.
flat anterior chamber	A potential complication of intraocular surgery characterized by the iris being in direct contact with the cornea and the virtual absence of aqueous in the anterior chamber.
fluorescein	A fluorescent dye.
footcandle	A measure of illumination. It is equal to a flux of one lumen radiated on a one square foot surface.
funduscopy	The process of looking at the fundus (the inside of the back of the eye).
genotype	The inherited gene combination.
giant cell	An inflammatory cell formed by the fusion of macrophages.
gonioscopy	The process of looking at the anterior chamber angle.
goniotomy	Opening a portion of the angle by incising a congenitally abnormal membrane that covers the trabecular meshwork.
hemoglobin	The reddish protein that carries oxygen in red blood cells.
hemolysis	The breakdown of red blood cells.
hemosiderosis	The tissue deposition of iron from degenerated red blood cells.

heterochromic — Mixed in color; used to describe two differently colored pupils.

hypermature lens — Usually denotes a cataract that is swollen and densely white.

hyperopic — Far-sighted, which implies a short eye ball.

hyperosmotic agent — A drug whose abnormally high osmotic force decreases the water content in many parts of the body, including the eye.

hyphema — Blood in the anterior chamber.

hypoxia — Poor oxygenation.

illumination — The light falling on an object (e.g. tangent screen, projection perimeter dome).

inferior — Downward in direction.

iridectomy — Excision of a piece of the iris.

iridocyclitis — Inflammation of both the iris and the ciliary body.

iridotomy — Making an incision in the iris.

iris — The anterior portion of the uvea that separates the anterior chamber from the lens and the posterior chamber. It is the colored part of the eye that has the pupil at its approximate center.

iris bombé — A forward bowing of the iris.

iris process — An extension of normal iris strands onto the scleral spur or the posterior trabecular meshwork.

isopter — A line of equal vision. It is formed by connecting the points on each meridian of the visual field where a target coming in from the periphery is first identified.

keratic — Corneal.

keratic precipitates — Deposits of cells on the corneal endothelium.

keratometer — An instrument to measure the curvature of the cornea.

kinetic perimetry — Visual field testing with a moving target whose size and luminance remain constant.

Krukenberg spindle — A linear collection of pigment on the corneal endothelium.

lacrimation — Tearing.

lamina	The perforated extension of the sclera through which optic nerve fibers leave the eye. It is located posterior to the optic nerve head and frequently can be seen normally at the base of the optic cup as a pale structure with darker dots scattered throughout.
laser	A device that transforms light into heat.
lens	The crystalline lens of the eye, whose physiologic changes in shape are responsible for focusing. As used in this text, "lens" always refers to crystalline lens unless indicated otherwise.
lens dislocation	Displacement of the lens due to ruptured zonules.
lens-induced	Caused by the lens; usually by its lysis, anaphylaxsis or dislocation.
local adaptation	The process whereby a particular locus on the retina becomes insensitive to a certain level of light intensity because of prolonged exposure.
longitudinal ciliary muscle	The portion of the ciliary body muscle that originates near the scleral equator and passes anteriorly to insert on the scleral spur.
luminance	The light emanating from an object.
macrophage	A wandering cell that ingests tissue debris when stimulated by inflammation.
meninges	The three membranes that cover the brain and spinal cord (dura mater, arachnoid, and pia mater).
meningioma	A benign tumor of the meninges; it can press on a portion of the nervous system and thereby destroy it.
metabolic acidosis	Acidification of the blood caused by a systemic metabolic abnormality, which can lead to deleterious alterations in the oxygenation of the brain.
methylcellulose	A viscid transparent solution used to keep air out of the interface between the cornea and a gonioscopic lens.

micrometer	A device for making very small measurements.
miosis	Making the pupil smaller.
miotic	A drug that constricts the pupil either by mimicking the parasympathetic effect of acetylcholine at the receptor site or by permitting more acetylcholine to accumulate there.
monocular	One-eyed.
morphology	Shape.
mydriasis	Making the pupil larger.
mydriatic	A drug that dilates the pupil by mimicking the sympathetic effect of norepinephrine at the receptor site.
myelinated	Refers to the white sheath that covers most of the nerves that arise from the brain or spinal cord.
myopic	Near-sighted; implies a long eye ball.
nasal	Toward the nose in direction.
nasal step	A visual field defect located at the nasal 180-degree meridian, and shaped like a stair-step.
neovascular	Made of newly formed blood vessels.
nerve rim overhang	A portion of the optic nerve head that hangs over a portion of the cup and partly hides it from view.
neurofibromatosis	A disease in which multiple small tumors are formed in many places throughout the body.
nodule	A small node.
nomogram	A table of precalculated mathematical values.
nuclear sclerosis	Opacification of the center of the lens, which causes it to change color gradually from yellow to brown.
occludable	Used to denote that the trabecular meshwork is occludable by iris.
occluded pupil	A pupil that is covered anteriorly by a membrane or by synechiae.
optic cup	The depression in the optic nerve head, which may be either normal or abnormal.
optic disc drusen	Hyaline bodies that are congenital in origin and are found in the anterior optic nerve.

optic nerve head, optic disc	The portion of the optic nerve (cranial nerve II) that can be seen ophthalmoscopically in the fundus of the eye. It is nearly round and pink and usually has a depression (or cup) in its center.
orbit	The bony structure surrounding the eye.
pantograph	A mechanical device used to reproduce exactly the location of the projection target in the perimeter's dome onto a piece of paper with a smaller scale. It consists of a framework of freely jointed metal rods set in the shape of a parallelogram.
paracentral	Near the center.
parasympathetic	A component of the autonomic nervous system. In the eye, it causes contraction of the iris sphincter with resultant miosis, and contraction of the ciliary muscle with resultant accommodation.
pericentral	Around the center.
periorbital	Around the orbit.
peripapillary	Around the papilla (optic nerve head).
periphery	The outside.
phacoanaphylactic	Hypersensitization to lens material.
phacolytic	Breakdown of the lens.
phakic	An eye possessing a crystalline lens.
photocoagulation	The process of coagulating tissue with the energy from light that has been transformed into heat by pigment cells.
photogrammetry	The process of making three dimensional maps from photographs.
photophobia	Abnormal sensitivity to light.
physiologic state	The normal condition.
pinocytosis	The ingestion of fluid by cells.
pituitary	A gland that is attached to the brain and secretes a number of important hormones; it is located near the junction of both optic nerves (the chiasm).
pituitary adenoma	A benign tumor of the pituitary gland; it can press on the chiasm and, thereby, destroy it.

plateau iris — A configuration of the iris that allows it to make an acute angle with the corneal periphery yet change direction to form a "plateau" centrally.

posterior — In back.

posterior chamber — The triangular space bounded by the posterior surface of the iris, the ciliary body and the anterior surface of the lens. It is the site where aqueous first enters the eye.

posterior synechiae — Fibrous scars of iridolenticular or iridovitreal adhesions.

prelaminar — In front of or anterior to the lamina.

prism — A glass or plastic lens that displaces the position of light rays.

profile — A side view (e.g. a cross section of the visual island).

projection perimeter — A hemispheric instrument with a white interior that is used for testing the visual field with a projected source of target light.

prone — Lying face down.

provocative test — A test to artificially provoke an elevation of intraocular pressure, which is a diagnostic sign of glaucoma.

pseudoexfoliation — The production of amorphous, dandruff-like material in the eye. It is called pseudoexfoliation owing to its superficial resemblance to true exfoliation of the lens capsule, which may, in fact, be part of the problem.

pseudofacility — A measurement of the volume of reduction of aqueous filtration each minute per mm Hg of intraocular pressure.

pupillary block — Obstruction of the forward transit of aqueous through the pupil.

quadrant — One of four equal parts.

radius — The straight-line distance from a point to a curve (e.g., from the center of a circle to its boundary).

retina — The sensory layer of the fundus of the eye whose rods and cones receive the visual impulse. Its nerve fibers come together at the optic disc to form the optic nerve.

psychophysical	Pertaining to the interaction between the psychological and physical.
retrolaminar	Behind or posterior to the lamina.
refraction	The process of determining or the actual measurement of the proper spectacle lenses that are needed to obtain the best possible vision.
rheostat	A device for regulating electric current.
rubeosis iridis	Formation of abnormal new blood vessels on the iris.
secluded pupil	A pupil that is bound completely by posterior synechiae.
Schlemm's canal	A circumferential (but irregular) channel for collecting aqueous that is buried in the sclera just outside of and connected to the trabecular meshwork, and just inside the episcleral veins.
Schwalbe's line	The line formed by the peripheral termination of Descemet's membrane of the cornea; it marks the anterior extent of the anterior chamber angle.
sclera	The white covering of the eye around its mid section and posterior extent.
scleral halo	A crescent of sclera at the border of the optic nerve head.
scleral rigidity	The ability of the sclera to withstand deformation.
scleral spur	The protrusion of white sclera into the anterior chamber angle, onto which the ciliary body inserts from behind.
sclerosis	Hardening.
scotoma	An abnormal blind area in the visual field.
spherical equivalent	The equivalent of the spectacle refraction expressed only as a sphere. To obtain it, take half of the cylinder and algebraically add it to the sphere.
sphincter	The circular iris muscle near the pupil that is primarily responsible for miosis.
static perimetry	Visual field testing with a stationary target whose luminance changes.
stereoscopic	Three-dimensional.

steroid	Used to imply a drug with anti-inflammatory capabilities; actually, a group name for a class of chemical compounds, which includes, among others, certain important hormones.
subthreshold	A stimulus strength below threshold.
superior	Up in direction.
suprathreshold	A stimulus strength greater than threshold.
sympathetic	A component of the autonomic nervous system. In the eye, it causes contraction of the iris dilator with resultant mydriasis.
syndrome	A specific group of signs or symptoms that comprise a particular disease.
tangent screen	A black square screen with a central fixation point for testing the visual field.
temporal	Toward the ear in direction.
threshold	The point at which a stimulus is just strong enough to be perceived.
tonography	A procedure for measuring the intraocular pressure and graphically recording it over time. From these readings, the coefficient of outflow can be calculated.
tonometer	An instrument to measure intraocular pressure.
trabecular meshwork	Multiple sheets of connective tissue with pores covered by endothelium through which the aqueous leaves the anterior chamber.
tumor	An abnormal growth of tissue which is not necessarily cancerous.
undermining	Erosion of the optic disc under a "shelf" of residual nerve tissue.
unilateral	One-sided.
uveitis	Inflammation of the uvea: iris, ciliary body, or choroid.
vacuole	A space in a cell.
vascular perfusion	The accessibility of blood or its products to the tissue.
vasculature	Blood vessel system.
visual field	The area and amount of vision perceived by the photo receptors outside of the fovea.

vitreous
: The gelatinous body between the retina and the lens.

zonules
: The "strings" of collagen that are attached to the lens around the equator and hold it to the ciliary body.

INDEX